Navigating the U.S. Hospice Maze

A short guide for community hospice physicians

Andy Arwari, MD, MS, FACP, FAAHPM, HMDC

Navigating the U.S. Hospice Maze. A short guide for community hospice physicians.

Andy Arwari MD, MS FACP, FAAHPM, HMDC

Copyright Year: 2023

Copyright Notice by Andy Arwari. All rights reserved

ISBN: 978-1-304-91705-8

The above information forms this copyright notice

To Nuria, Julia, and Alex, the stars that light up my universe. Thank you for your love and support through all my crazy endeavors.

To all the compassionate human beings who selflessly dedicate themselves to work in hospice care so that others may transition peacefully.

Acknowledgment

I wanted to thank Judi Chase, APRN, Ann Flanagan Petry, LCSW, and Rev Jennifer Rund- Scott, M. Div. BCC, my original interdisciplinary palliative care team, for their support and encouragement. I would not be in the hospice and palliative care field today if it were not for the example of interdisciplinary teamwork and collaboration I experienced early on in my career. Because of that experience and example, I advocate and continue to support the interdisciplinary team approach to care. Interdisciplinary team care should not only apply to hospice and palliative care but should be the prevailing model throughout our entire healthcare system.

I am extending my gratitude and appreciation to all my present hospice interdisciplinary team members who continue to make the journey possible. Your unwavering commitment to providing high-quality end-of-life care is a constant source of personal motivation to continue improving the provision of hospice and palliative care in an equitable, compassionate, and interdisciplinary way.

Table of Contents

Acknowledgment	iv
Introduction	8
1. Background on Hospice	11
2. Hospital-Centric Care	15
3. How Does Hospice Fit into Medicare?	19
4. Death Denying Culture	26
5. Advance Care Planning	36
6. Time for Hospice	46
7. Preparing for the Hospice Talk	50
8. Presenting Hospice to Patients	54
9. Prognostication	58
10. The Imminent Patient	72
11. Prognostication Funnel	78
12. Code of Federal Regulations	82
13. Medicare Administrative Contractor	99

14. Patients Stopping Hospice Care 109
15. Discharge from Hospice 113
16. The Hospice Team 123
17. Hospice Medications 128
18. The Four Levels of Hospice 134
19. Hospice Funding 143
20. The Hospice Patient and the ED 155
21. Primary Care and other Physicians 161
22. Advice about Pain Management 168
23. The Agitated Hospice Patient 180
24. Hospice Program Quality Measures 187
25. Hospice Survey 195
26. The Elephant in the Room. Medical Assistance in Dying (MAiD) 199
27. Death Certificates 203
28. Bereavement and Condolences 209
29. Hospice Advocacy in the Community 212
30. Final Thoughts 220
    Index 223

Introduction

I wrote this short guide colloquially as I want this to be practical advice. This guide aims to help non-hospice and palliative care specialist-trained physicians gain their bearings while working in hospice. I point them toward resources to help them expand their knowledge of hospice and integrate it into the interdisciplinary team model necessary to provide excellent end-of-life care. I have used the term interdisciplinary team in this guide instead of interdisciplinary group. A team has shared goals, holds each other accountable, and succeeds or fails together[1]. As physicians we are used to working independently, however, in hospice, we must relinquish hierarchy and integrate into the team to meet the patient's needs.

Non-fellowship-trained community physicians should know they can be officially recognized for their skill and competency through the Hospice Medical Director Certification (HMDC) board exam. Hopefully, after reading this guide, more community physicians practicing hospice will continue to expand their knowledge of hospice care and seek recognition through board certification.

As per the National Hospice and Palliative Care Organization (NHPCO) 2022 fact sheets, over 5000 hospices are operating presently in the United States [2]. Most physicians providing supervision and care to hospice patients in the U.S. are not palliative specialty-trained physicians, yet these physicians offer the best possible end-of-life care.

By 2030, one out of every five Americans is projected to be 65 years older and Medicare eligible, especially Medicare Part A[3]. As per the 2022 NHPCO fact and figure sheet, 1.7 million Medicare beneficiaries were enrolled in hospice in 2020 [2]. This figure translates into approximately half of all beneficiaries who died in 2020 using their hospice benefit. Ten thousand patients are entering Medicare each day[3], so we should expect hospice utilization to increase yearly. Currently, one-fourth of Medicare spending is for patients in their last year of life [4]. The lion's share of this spending is on hospitalizations, procedures, interventions, and rehabilitation intent. Later in the guide, you will see the billions of dollars the U.S. government spends on each part of Medicare (Table 6). We are the only country in the world to fully fund an end-of-life service through federal tax collection. There are several questions we should be asking ourselves. Do we allocate sufficient resources to end-of-life care? Given the projected increase in expected hospice care utilization, are we prepared for future service needs? Hopefully, we will work on ensuring sufficient resources are in place to provide equitable and quality end-of-life care.

References

1. Asana. Group vs. Team: What's the Difference? • Asana. Asana. Published October 14, 2021. https://asana.com/resources/group-vs-team

2. NHPCO Facts and Figures 2022 Edition. December 2022. https://www.nhpco.org/wp-content/uploads/NHPCO-Facts-Figures-2022.pdf Accessed June 3, 2023

3. Goldhirsch S. *Geriatric Palliative Care*. Oxford University Press; 2014.

4. Sagha Zadeh R, Eshelman P, Setla J, Sadatsafavi H. Strategies to Improve Quality of Life at the End of Life: Interdisciplinary Team Perspectives. *American Journal of Hospice and Palliative Medicine®*. 2017;35(3):411-416. doi:https://doi.org/10.1177/1049909117711997

1.
Background on Hospice

Wisdom begins in wonder.

Socrates

Hospices were formally established in the 12th century to offer the homeless and frail refuge. By the 19th century, most hospices were supported and staffed by Catholic, Anglican, and Methodist nuns who cared for society's less fortunate people [1]. Dr. Cicely Saunders, a British physician, is credited with modernizing hospice care [1,2]. She started her healthcare career in 1940, earning a nursing degree [1,2]. She then returned to school and earned a degree in medical social work from Oxford University [1]. She furthered her education by completing an M.D. in 1958. After completing her Medical Doctor degree, she completed a six-year research fellowship at St. Joseph's Hospice in England [1]. Her unique background allowed her to develop the total pain framework and model the holistic team-based approach to provide end-of-life care [2]. Dr. Saunders went on to found St. Christopher's Hospice in London, a center of excellence for end-of-life care where innovative treatments would be pioneered, and future hospice and palliative care luminaries would receive training. Dr. Saunders visited the U.S. in the 60s and catalyzed the modern hospice movement. Along with other visionaries like Florance Wald and Dr. Elizabeth Kübler Ross [4], the hospice movement would grow locally in many communities around the United States.

Because of the recognized patient benefits and the cost savings to Medicare, hospice became integrated into our healthcare system through the inception of the Medicare Hospice Benefit in 1983 under the Tax Equity and Fiscal Responsibility Act of 1982 [5]. The United States is the only country in the world where hospice is integrated into its healthcare delivery system through the Medicare program and, as such, receives funding from the federal government. In the U.S., our Code of Federal Regulations establishes, based on Cicely Saunders' modern hospice care model, that end-of-life care be provided by an interdisciplinary care team [3].

Unfortunately, many U.S. citizens are unaware of how this critical benefit is funded or that it is indeed a benefit. Hospice continues to be viewed as a medical decision often offered to patients when conventional therapies no longer provide any improvement or benefit to a patient in their disease course. As hospice physicians, we need to be able to explain the benefits of hospice enrollment to patients and families as well as educate our fellow clinicians. We need to help ease the transition to end-of-life by emphasizing that hospice care is not abandonment or rationing of care.

References

1. Vanderpool HY. *Palliative Care: The 400-Year Quest for a Good Death*. Mcfarland & Company, Inc., Publishers; 2015.

2. Connor SR. *Hospice and Palliative Care*. Third Edition. Taylor & Francis; 2017.

3. Code of Federal Regulations Title 42 Public Health. Office of the Federal Register;2017 Accessed June 2, 2023

4. Buck, J. "I am Willing to Take the Risk", Politics, Policy, and the Translation of the Hospice Ideal. ("'I am willing to take the risk': politics, policy and the ...") J Clin Nurs. 2009(18)19: 2700-2709. doi: 10.1111/j.1365-2702.2009.02890.x. Available at: http://survey.hshsl.umaryland.edu/?url=http://search.ebscohost.com/login.aspx?direct=true&db=cmedm&AN=19744021&site=eds-live

5. Kobayashi R, McAllister CA. Similarities and Differences in Perspectives on Interdisciplinary Collaboration Among Hospice Team Members. *American Journal of Hospice and Palliative Medicine®*.2013;31(8):825-832. doi:https://doi.org/10.1177/1049909113503706

2.
Hospital-Centric Care

Harmony makes small things grow, lack of it makes great things decay.
                                    Sallust

Would it surprise you to learn that the U.S. has a hospital-centric healthcare delivery model? This hospital-centric care model originates in the Hospital Survey and Construction Act of 1946 or the Hill-Burton Act. The Act aimed to survey state hospitals and health facilities and determine where additional facilities were needed to ensure access to healthcare [1]. It was also intended to correlate and integrate hospitals and the public health service so that all parts of the country would receive adequate health services. The Hill-Burton Act did expand the U.S. healthcare systems infrastructure between 1947 and 1971, but it did so by directing more than 70% of the allotted federal dollars to build acute-short-term hospitals which made up 54% of the infrastructure projects. Only 6% of federal funding was directed to outpatient facilities which accounted for 10% of the overall projects, and only 3% went to build public health centers [1]. The result of how the money was spent is that infrastructure was built to favor and support acute care (See Table 1).

Table 1. Breakdown of federal dollars spent on U.S infrastructure between 1947-1971 [1].

Type of Facility	% of Project	% Federal Funding
Acute –Short Term Hospitals	54%	71%
Long Term Hospitals including nursing home and chronic Hospitals	16%	14%
Outpatient facilities	10%	6%
Public Health Centers	12%	3%

Another important factor that affected how we provide healthcare in the U.S. was that the physician workforce shifted towards specialists. In 1949 more than half of the U.S physician workforce was made up of general practitioners. Today roughly 70% of the U.S. physician workforce are specialists that work for healthcare systems tied to acute care hospitals where highly specialized technology-driven care is provided [1]. Surprised? We built hospitals which in turn promoted specialist care. We prioritize acute care and procedures over preventive health and social programs.

Here lies the reason why the majority of Americans seek their care in the hospital. The emergency department is the gateway to acute care hospitals. We cannot blame patients for seeking ED and acute care hospital care. Our healthcare system in the U.S. was built to favor this model. We should also acknowledge that we need more primary care physicians. In the U.S., primary care physicians are at a disadvantage regarding numbers, resources, and access to advanced technological care. We need to stop thinking that access to care can be shifted to outpatient physicians, who make up less than half of the U.S. physician workforce. Until we can fix the workforce imbalance, we will continue to see overutilization of acute care resources. Another downstream effect of the primary care workforce shortage is that there are not enough clinicians dedicating the necessary time to explore patients' wishes, values, and preferences. There is a general belief in the medical community that primary care physicians are the ones that are responsible for addressing advance care planning with patients. We need to change that mindset. All clinicians interacting with a patient must become competent in addressing the patient's wishes, values, and preferences. If we do not change this model, we cannot expect to make progress towards ensuring that advance care planning is completed for most patients, if not all of them.

Reference

1. Ameringer C. *US Health Policy and Health Care Delivery, Doctors, Reformers and Entrepreneurs*. Cambridge University Press; 2018

3.
How Does Hospice Fit into Medicare?

Change is not made without inconvenience, even from worse to better.
                    Richard Hooker

Medicare came into existence in 1965 to cover the healthcare needs of the elderly who for the most part did not have healthcare insurance coverage before Medicare. There are four parts to Medicare; A, B, C, and D. Medicare Parts A and B were the original Medicare. Part C and D were introduced in 2003 with the Medicare Modernization Act under the George W. Bush administration. I will focus here on Medicare Part A and mention a couple of things related to Medicare Part B and D later on when we discuss how patients in hospice may continue to see non-hospice physicians and how they can continue to receive non-hospice-related medications.

Medicare Part C is Medicare Advantage or Medicare covered by private insurance companies. I will not address Medicare Advantage but you should know that there will likely be changes coming in the future that will impact hospice and palliative care.

Confusing right? Imagine patients and their families having to navigate the bureaucracy of Medicare. You can see why the word maze is included in the title of this book.

Let's look at the basic breakdown of Medicare (Figure 1).

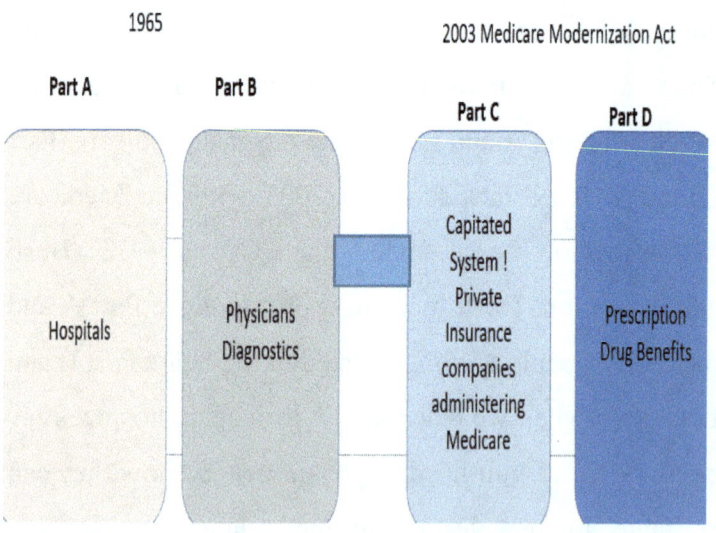

Figure 1. Breakdown of Medicare by Parts.

Medicare Part A covers hospitalizations, skilled nursing facilities for rehabilitation and restoration intents, home health care, dialysis, AND **hospice**.

Who is eligible for Medicare Part A?

- o At age 65, anyone eligible for Social Security is AUTOMATICALLY enrolled in Medicare Part A whether they are retired or not. To qualify a person has to have paid into Social Security for 10 years.

- o People under the age of 65 who are TOTALLY and PERMANENTLY disabled may enroll in Medicare Part A after receiving Social Security disability benefits for 24 months.

- o People with amyotrophic lateral disease or end-stage renal disease (ESRD) requiring dialysis are eligible for Medicare Part A immediately. They are the exception to the above and do not have to wait 24 months.

Medicare Part A is funded through payroll taxes.

- Employers and employees each pay Medicare the equivalent of 1.45% of payroll taxes.
- If you are self-employed, you pay 2.9% of your payroll towards the Medicare Part A fund.
- In 2010 the Affordable Care Act (ACA) changed the rate for higher income brackets. If you make more than $200,000 or more than $250,000 joint filing, you pay 2.35% and not 1.45% of payroll tax to fund the Medicare Part A fund.

When a patient has reached the end stage of their chronic progressive disease and is more likely than not to have a life expectancy of six months or less they become eligible for hospice.

What happens here is that Medicare Part A and all the services under it become hospice if the patient elects their end-of-life care!

Think of it this way for simplification purposes:

A becomes H

For clarification, there is no Medicare Part H. This is only to help you understand what happens to Medicare Part A services when a patient chooses their hospice benefit.

I do want to address dialysis. If electing hospice for a primary terminal diagnosis of ESRD, the patient is not eligible to continue dialysis because it is housed under Medicare Part A. Fair? In my humble opinion no! A patient that has another chronic progressive terminal disease can still be eligible for hospice and not have to choose to forgo dialysis. This is a loophole that I hope one day will be closed. Patients with ESRD should not be made to choose to stop dialysis so they can receive hospice services. The median survival after stopping dialysis is 7-10 days [2].

Let's look at an example:

Mr. North is an ESRD patient who has been on dialysis for the last 4 years. He has lost weight due to poor appetite and has been hospitalized twice this year for dialysis catheter-related sepsis. He is struggling to complete *all his activities of daily living (ADLs) and needs his son's assistance. He recently visited his primary care physician who recommended a hospice consult. He is evaluated by hospice and is informed that he is eligible but needs to stop dialysis. Prognosis is discussed with the patient and son. Mr. North declines hospice because he is hoping to live long enough to see his grandson's graduation in two months. A 7-10 days prognosis is not acceptable to him at this time.*

Is it fair to tell a dialysis-dependent patient that they can only access their benefit by stopping dialysis? Mr. North may not live to see his grandson's graduation but he and his family will benefit tremendously from receiving hospice care, especially in light of his evident decline.

We do not require patients to be DNR to access hospice but we require ESRD patients to stop dialysis if they wish to enroll in hospice. Food for thought.

References

1. Bodenheimer T, Grumbach K. *Understanding Health Policy A Clinical Approach*. Eight Edition. Lange; 2020

2. O'Connor NR, Dougherty M, Harris PS, Casarett DJ. Survival after dialysis discontinuation and hospice enrollment for ESRD. *Clin J Am Soc Nephrol*. 2013;8(12):2117-2122. doi:10.2215/CJN.04110413

4.
Death Denying Culture

Ignorance is the soil in which belief in miracles grows.
Robert Ingersoll

We live in a death-denying culture that has placed high hopes on medical technology to extend life. In the 1940s, we identified blood compatibility, which led to the ability to transfuse blood. Antibiotics were discovered, which increased our capabilities to fight infections. In the 1950s, the first kidney was transplanted, and shortly after that, immunosuppressive medications were developed, which reduced organ transplant rejections [1]. The iron lung was developed in the 1950s from which evolved our modern ventilators and our ability to provide assisted respiratory support. Cardiac procedures such as CPR and coronary bypass surgery were also developed in the late

1950s [1]. As a consequence of these new therapies and interventions intensive care units and coronary care units were established in hospitals all across the U.S. [1].

Medicine has had a fantastic expansion of diagnostic and treatment capabilities in the last 80 years. In our quest to expand our capabilities to improve the human condition, we have lost sight that medical care should focus on promoting and enhancing the quality of life. We are mortal beings, and we cannot avoid death. We should educate our patients on their diagnosis, treatment options, and prognosis.

Next time you evaluate a patient in your clinic or hospital, closely examine the patient's problem list. Do they have a chronic progressive terminal disease? Take a close look at the patient's medication list and any other treatment they have received or are receiving for their disease. Ask the patient how the medications and interventions have impacted their quality of life. Chronic diseases such as cancer, end-organ failure, and dementia follow a specific trajectory (See Fig. 2). A good exercise is to draw the corresponding graph of your patient's chronic terminal disease trajectory before moving forward. The star on the graphs would indicate the point in a patient's disease trajectory where they would benefit from hospice. Where do you think the patient in front of you is on their disease trajectory? Is it possible that they are indeed at the star or near the star?

Graph 1. Patient with cancer

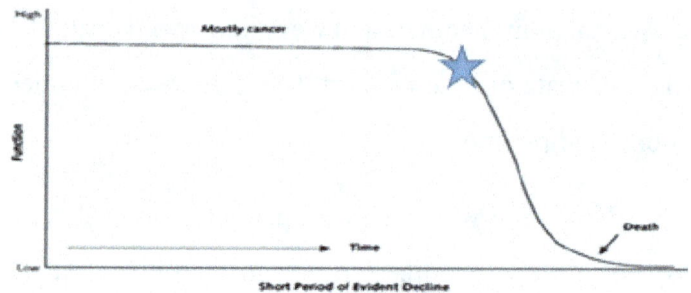

Graph 2. Patient with end organ failure (Heart, Lung, Kidney, Liver)

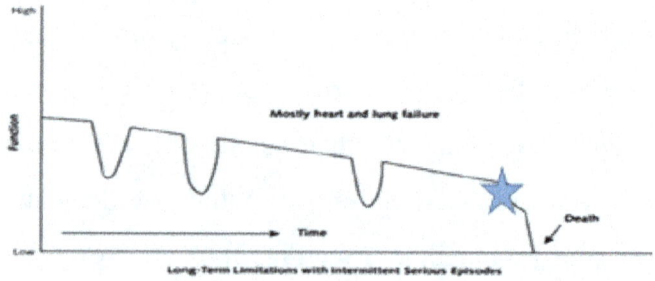

Graph 3. Patient with dementia

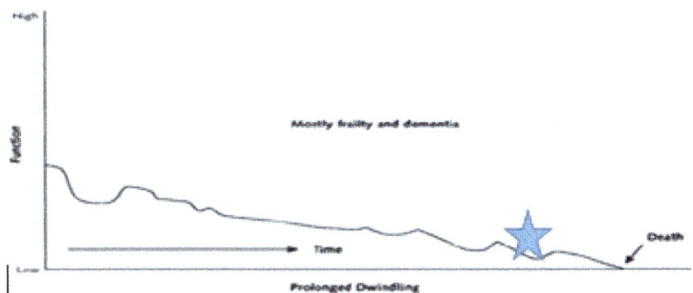

Figure 2. Disease trajectories. Permission granted to use and adapt figure from RAND WP-137 [2].

Let's look at some examples.

Mrs. Jones is an 82-year-old female patient with stage 4 colon cancer. She was able to get out of bed with some assistance and needed help from her daughter to dress and bathe but could eat on her own. She developed a cough which was thought to be bronchitis and had a rapid decline.

Mrs. Jones would likely follow graph number one.

Mr. Green is a 76-year-old patient with systolic heart failure. His latest ejection fraction(EF) was 15%. He has an automatic implantable cardiac defibrillator

(AICD). He is short of breath all the time and has just returned from the hospital. It would be his third hospitalization for congestive heart failure(CHF) exacerbation in the last two months.

Mr. Green would likely follow graph #2 as would any patient with an organ failure.

Mrs. Adams is an 86-year-old female patient who was diagnosed with Alzheimer's disease 12 years ago. She has also had labile essential hypertension for the last 10 years and is on three different antihypertensive medications. She has suffered 2 cerebral vascular accidents (CVA)for which she has been hospitalized. She is no longer able to do any of her activities of daily living.

She would likely follow graph #3.

As you can see not all patients with chronic progressive diseases will follow the same trajectory. Chances are that a patient has more than one chronic progressive disease. A good starting point for self-reflection is to draw your patient's graph out and be able to share it with the patient and their loved ones to help them visualize the trajectory their disease will likely follow and where they may be in that trajectory. Hopefully, this will lead to an open and transparent conversation about issues such as why medications or procedures they may have had may no longer control their symptoms as they once did. It is an opportunity to discuss future care and allow patients to plan for that future by completing advance directives.

Has the patient completed an advance directive?

Mrs. Applebaum is a 75-year-old female patient with long-standing systolic congestive heart failure. She had an echocardiogram last month during hospitalization for acute chronic congestive heart failure (CHF) exacerbation, which showed her ejection fraction to be 25%. Her most recent ECHO from a year ago showed an EF of 35%. Mrs. Applebaum was scheduled to follow up both with her primary care physician and her cardiologist after being discharged. She became severely short of breath and her family called 911. Upon arrival emergency medical services (EMS) found her to be tachypnea and her oxygen saturation at 76%. She was intubated in the field and taken to the emergency department (ED). She was found to be hypotensive and was started on norepinephrine and broad-spectrum antibiotics. She is also found to be in acute on chronic renal failure. She is admitted to the intensive care unit (ICU) where she continued to receive mechanical ventilation and she is started on ultrafiltration dialysis for acute renal failure.

She does not have any advance directives. She has never discussed her wishes, values, and preferences for healthcare with her family. The ICU team has kept her family informed and has explained that she has not shown any signs of improvement with the interventions provided. Two days later Mrs. Applebaum expires in the ICU while tethered to an endotracheal tube, nasogastric tube, and a left subclavian triple lumen central line.

Is this how she would want to spend her final moments? Was she comfortable? In case you are wondering, if reviewing her medical records, we would have concluded that Mrs. Applebaum was at the end of the CHF trajectory if we had graphed her disease out, and she could have elected hospice care if presented with the option after her last hospitalization. A missed opportunity to have a discussion about her wishes and values and update her preferences before she was discharged home from her recent hospital stay before returning and being admitted to the ICU.

Most Americans would like to die at home, surrounded by their loved ones, and not in a sterile ICU setting, hooked up to tubes and devices and alone. Unfortunately, only 1 in 3 Americans have completed any type of advance directive [3]. If incapacitated, a patient who has not let their wishes and values be known may be subjected to interventions they may not have elected to have if given the option. Worst of all, there may be ambiguity presented to a patient's proxy or family on what the advanced treatment modalities or trials may be able to accomplish. In the heat of a crisis, no one reflects on where the patient may be on their disease trajectory curve or where they may have advanced due to the acute decline that brought them into the hospital. Families may feel conflicted and confused about forgoing treatment and therefore, have their loved ones admitted to ICU to receive advanced therapies and interventions such as mechanical ventilation, dialysis, and artificial nutrition and hydration.

As I mentioned initially, our physician workforce has shifted towards specialists. We cannot continue to believe that only primary care physicians can discuss advance care planning. How about palliative care? Not every hospital in the U.S. has a palliative care service; if there is one, it may not be fully staffed or be available 7 days a week. Here is an opportunity for hospital administrators to establish palliative care programs in their healthcare systems. These programs need to be staffed adequately to function as interdisciplinary palliative care teams and they should focus on allowing the palliative care team to be integrated early into the care of hospitalized patients.

In 1990, Congress passed the Patient Self-Determination Act that directs any healthcare facility receiving Medicare or Medicaid funding to make advance care planning discussions available to patients [4]. We should ask ourselves who is providing this education to patients and families. Is it just asking on admission to a healthcare facility, especially a hospital, if a patient wants to be full code or DNR, fulfilling the Patient Self-Determination Act requirement?

It will take all of us, irrespective of our role in our healthcare system, to raise awareness about advance care planning and actively address the low completion rate of advance care planning.

References

1. Vanderpool HY. *Palliative Care: The 400-Year Quest for a Good Death.* Mcfarland & Company, Inc., Publishers; 2015.

2. Lynn J, Adamson D. *Living Well at the End of Life: Adapting Health Care to Serious Chronic Illness in Old Age.*; 2003. doi:https://doi.org/10.7249/wp137

3. Yadav KN, Gabler NB, Cooney E, et al. Approximately one in three US adults completes any type of advance directive for end-of-life care. *Health Affairs.* 2017;36(7):1244-1251. doi:https://doi.org/10.1377/hlthaff.2017.0175

4. H.R.5067 Patient Self Determination Act 1990. Congress.Gov https://www.congress.gov/bill/101st-congress/house-bill/5067 Accessed July 12, 2023

5.
Advance Care Planning

The reward of a thing well done is having done it.

Ralph Waldo Emerson

Advance care planning (ACP) is the inherent responsibility we as clinicians hold to ensure we provide our patients with medical care according to their wishes, values, and preferences.

The forms used to document advance care planning complement clinicians' thorough, compassionate, and realistic discussions with their patients. Handing or mailing these forms to patients and expecting them to complete them defeats the purpose of advance care planning. These forms by themselves are never a substitute for the communication that should be occurring between clinicians and patients.

Advance care directive is an umbrella term under which we find multiple forms that can express a patient's wishes and values. I will list the most common forms you should be familiar with.

Living Will: Legal document directing a physician to treatments a patient may want or not want and can specify conditions when to apply. They may be very broad and generic. We risk interjecting our own interpretation bias, especially when the language is ambiguous.

Durable power of attorney for health care: Legal document naming a proxy, surrogate, or agent that will make medical decisions on behalf of a patient if the patient is incapacitated. It only takes effect if patients can no longer express their wishes, values, and preferences. This is why assessing and determining if a patient has medical decision-making capacity is essential. A proxy or surrogate would only make decisions on behalf of a patient when we determine that a patient lacks medical decision-making capacity.

You can use the U-ARE criteria: Understanding, Appreciation, Rationality, and Expression of Choice to assess decision-making capacity [1].

Let's look at an example:*Mrs. Ramirez is a 72-year-old female patient admitted to your hospice a month ago with a primary diagnosis of End Stage Liver Disease. Her son calls to speak to you and mentions that his mother would like to have a knee replacement surgery that had been discussed a year ago with an Orthopedic surgeon the patient had been referred to for an evaluation.*

You visit the patient and find her to be confused. You use the U-ARE criteria. You determine that she is not able to understand the intent of a knee replacement surgery. She cannot appreciate either the benefits or the risks. She cannot rationalize her request. You have enough to determine that the patient lacks medical decision capacity and could not, therefore, consent to the procedure.

Your next step is to educate her son who is listed as the healthcare proxy that the patient is not able to make complex decisions such as consenting for the procedure. You will also need to educate the son as to why such an intervention would likely detract from the patient's quality of life and would not be consistent with a hospice plan of care. As bizarre as this scenario may sound, these situations do happen in hospice.

Recall that physicians determine decision capacity and not competence. A way I remind myself of this is to state it as medical decision-making capacity. Competency is a legal determination. Capacity if a medical determination. There is no medical competency [2].

Do not resuscitate order (DNR): Often confused as an order not to provide medical care. DNR is only applicable if the patient's heartbeat and breathing stop! It means that the patient has elected not to undergo cardio pulmonary resuscitation (CPR). PATIENTS DO NOT HAVE TO BE DNR TO ENROLL IN HOSPICE! Read again. Why is that? Hospice is an entitlement program. A benefit cannot be conditioned on the patient's choice of code status. Both hospice care and code status are a patient's choice! Read again. Requesting that a patient be DNR before proceeding to enroll them in hospice would violate federal statutes.

When addressing code status and any other intervention our job as hospice clinicians is to make sure it is an informed choice based on skillful, transparent, and compassionate education. We should not address CPR discussions with "we will crack all your ribs." We should explore what the patient understands about their disease, where they understand they are in their disease trajectory, and what they hope for when undergoing an attempt at CPR. We can describe the procedures honestly and compassionately and explore if they make sense to the patient. Instead of explaining the cracking of ribs, we can emphasize that none of these procedures will change the prognosis should the patient be fortunate to survive. Would death in an intensive care unit or long-term care facility (LTAC) be acceptable to the patient?

Do not hospitalize: Some patients may have already decided that they would not wish to return to the hospital.

ICU care should also be explicitly discussed with patients. Most patients and families have likely never visited the restricted environment of a hospital's intensive care unit. Is this really how your patient wants to spend their final moments? Hooked up to machines, tubes with flashing lights, and constant beeping?

Image 1: Intensive Care Unit.

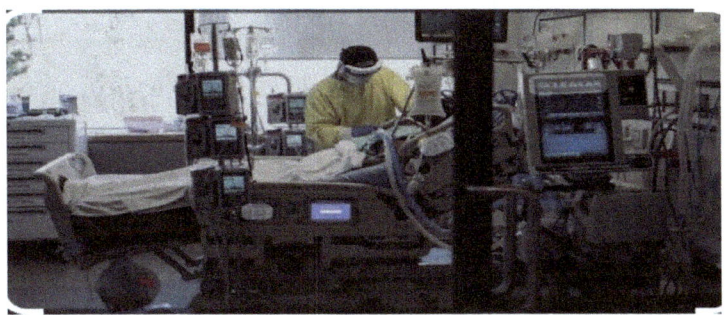

They likely do not fully understand what they may be in for. We should explain what therapies and interventions may be provided in the ICU and explain that these interventions may prolong life but they will ultimately not reverse the end stage of a chronic progressive disease. We should explore if a patient values quality over quantity and educate them on what any intervention will likely provide.

Physician orders for life-sustaining treatment (POLST) and Medical orders for life-sustaining treatment (MOLST) forms: These forms allow us to explore the scope of acceptable treatments and interventions a patient may accept. For example, a patient may agree to receive antibiotics and iv fluids in a hospital but not wish for care to be escalated to ICU care. They may not wish to consider dialysis should they be determined to have renal failure. Artificial nutrition and hydration (ANH) should also be discussed. A patient may clearly state that if no longer able to eat through the natural route they would not wish to have a percutaneous gastrostomy tube (PEG) placed.

I am including the link to the National Institute of Aging resource on Advance Care Planning in reference [3]. I recommend you check it out. You will find a link to the Advance Care Planning, Conversation Guide that you can download for free. You can share this resource with your community physician colleagues.

Perhaps the most important point of discussion in advance care planning is the opportunity to educate about hospice. Explore and educate patients and families about their understanding of this benefit and if they would consider it if they were ever provided a terminal prognosis. It may also be helpful to provide patients and families with written information about hospice services for them to read and reference. As a hospice physician, you need to be able to speak about hospice care and dispel all the misinformation and misconceptions that are still out at large in our communities.

Even if these forms have been filled out before hospice admission, ask the patient or their proxy if what is stated and reflected in the forms is still consistent with a patient's wishes, values, and preferences.

Let me share an example:

Mr. Martinez is a 78-year-old male patient who was hospitalized for acute shortness of breath. He has advanced systolic heart failure. He had an ECHO which showed his EF to be 15%. He was treated with a Lasix infusion and was followed by cardiology. A year ago Mr. Martinez had an AICD implanted. Despite diuresing more than 4 liters, he remains short of breath at rest. The cardiology team informs the hospitalist that there are no further Guideline Directed Therapies that can be offered. Hospice is recommended and the patient and family agree.

Due to ongoing shortness of breath, he is directly transferred upon hospice admission to your inpatient hospice unit to address and alleviate his shortness of breath. Upon admission, his records state that he is a full code.

You complete the hospice admission and as part of your history and physical, address ethical and legal issues. You specifically ask the patient about his advance directives in the presence of his proxy, his daughter Mariana. The patient informs you that he does not want to be kept alive by any artificial means. Mariana confirms that her Dad has stated this since the AICD implantation a year ago. The code status is updated to DNR for Mr. Martinez.

It would have been easy to assume that the patient was a full code. He was after all transferred from the hospital to the inpatient hospice unit as such. It should never be assumed that advance care planning has been previously or completely addressed before admission to hospice. As you take the time to know your patient and their family, it is important to specifically and explicitly address advance care planning.

References

1. Palmer BW, Harmell AL. Assessment of Healthcare Decision-making Capacity. *Arch Clin Neuropsychol.* 2016;31(6):530-540. doi:10.1093/arclin/acw051Capacity v.

2. Competency and Why it Matters | MIEC. https://www.miec.com/knowledge-library/capacity-v-competency-and-why-it-matters/

3. Advance Care Planning: Advance Directives for Health Care. National Institute on Aging. https://www.nia.nih.gov/health/advance-care-planning-advance-directives-health-care Accessed June 5, 2023

6.
Time for Hospice

> *There are two sides to every question.*
>
> Protagoras

What terminal progressive disease does your patient have? Your patient will follow one of the three disease trajectory graphs in Figure 2. After finding the most appropriate graph, ask yourself if you would be surprised if this patient were to pass away in the next year? Would it be reasonable for you to think this patient has, indeed, a prognosis of six months or less?

Some indicators can help you answer the six-month prognosis. Start by questioning the activities of daily living (ADLs) [1]. Can the patient independently perform any of the six activities of daily living: eating, bathing, dressing, transferring, toileting, walking, or moving around? Have there been changes in their ability to perform their ADLs? Do they need assistance, and to what degree?

What about the patient's nutrition? How many meals a day is the patient eating? How much are they eating? Has there been weight loss? How much and in what time frame? Are there signs the patient can no longer swallow their food? What about the patient's cognition? Can the patient still speak? Can their speech be understood? Can the patient answer questions? Can they direct care? How much time are they sleeping in a 24 hours period? Here is a perfect opportunity to assess medical decision-making capacity.

Hopefully, you can determine if hospice may be right at this time for your patient. Figure 3 below is to help you visualize the observed and expected decline with a likely six-month prognosis if the disease runs its natural course.

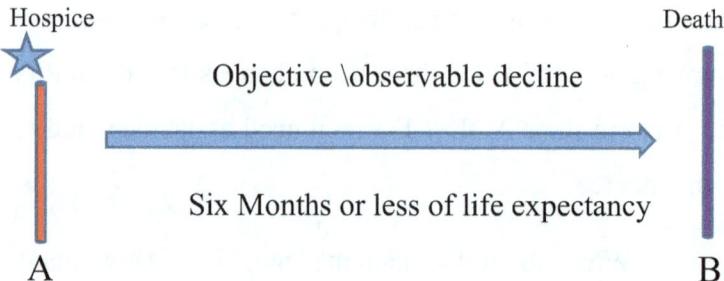

Figure 3. Distance illustrating end-stage disease to death.

Point A would be your star on your patient's disease trajectory graph (Fig.2) where the patient would be eligible for hospice. Point B would be when the patient is likely to pass away if we provide a six-month prognosis (Fig.3).

You determine that your patient is hospice eligible. You can take the opportunity to discuss with them access to their hospice benefit. By doing so you are allowing them and their family time to prepare for end-of-life and allow them to receive the necessary support they will need to maximize quality of life.

As you are introducing hospice care, I would remind you to emphasize to the patient and their families that it is a benefit and that it is their choice to elect it. You are simply making them aware of the benefit and can help facilitate their access by certifying them.

Reference

1. Activities of Daily Living – CMS.gov 2008. https://www.cms.gov/research-statistics-data-and-systems/research/mcbs/downloads/2008_appendix_b.pdf Accessed June 6, 2023

7.

Preparing for the Hospice Talk

> *Respond intelligently even to unintelligent treatment.*
>
> Lao Tzu

Be prepared to have a conversation about hospice with patients and families. I am listing below the important talking points you will need to address for the conversation to be as meaningful and helpful for the patient.

1. The patient understands they have a chronic progressive terminal disease. This is a sensitive discussion and where clinicians should use the SPIKES protocol [1].

- S – Setting. Make sure the discussion will be held in a location that is private, and comfortable. Make sure there is water, glasses, and tissues
- P- Perception. What do the patient and family know? Explore, be silent allow them to offer their view on what is happening.
- I- Invitation. Ask the patient or primary caregiver what they would like to know.
- K- Knowledge. Explain what is happening. Draw the graph. Tell them what can be done and how this will help the patient.
- E- Emotions. Respect feelings, and acknowledge them. Respond with compassion.
- S- Summarize. Recap the discussion. Make sure that the patient and/or family express an adequate

understanding of what has just been discussed.
2. The patient is at a stage of their disease where they will not benefit from disease-directed care.
3. They can now access their Medicare hospice entitlement program. Explain how this has been funded by them. There is no cost to the patient and family once the benefit has been accessed. Explain how this ties into Medicare Part A. Hopefully you are now equipped to do so!
4. Educate the patient and their family on how hospice will focus on providing them the quality of life for whatever time they may have left and will also focus on their families.
5. Highlight how they will now have a whole interdisciplinary care team. Mention which specific disciplines will provide care and their roles.
6. Explain how care will be provided mainly in the home, and patients will be provided the necessary equipment and medications to address their end-of-life needs.

7. The MOST important is to make the point: IT IS THE PATIENT'S CHOICE to enroll in their BENEFIT!

What we never want to convey is that:

1. We, clinicians, are choosing hospice for the patient.
2. We are directly or indirectly communicating to the patient that there is nothing left to do.

Reference

1. Wittenberg E, Ferrell BR, Goldsmith J, Smith T, Ragan SL, Handzo GF. *Textbook of Palliative Care Communication*. Oxford University Press; 2016.

8.
Presenting Hospice to Patients

> *In some cases, silence is dangerous.*
>
> Saint Ambrose

Mrs. Smith is a 77-year-old female with stage D heart failure. She is dyspneic at rest despite wearing 2 liters of oxygen continuously. She requires assistance with all her ADLs. Her appetite is poor, and she has lost 15 lbs. since you last saw her in the clinic a month ago. She is disoriented to time but will answer simple questions. Her daughter is with her. She has been hospitalized twice last month for acute on chronic exacerbation of systolic congestive heart failure exacerbation. During her last hospitalization, she was seen by the inpatient palliative care service, and hospice was suggested.

This is a typical scenario that occurs each day across the U.S. Most primary care physicians are tasked with having this crucial conversation about hospice but feel overwhelmed due to time constraints and being uncomfortable for fear they are conveying giving up on their patients.

The unfortunate, unspoken truth is that delaying or avoiding this conversation robs the patient of a benefit! Let's look at where hospice fits into the care of a patient like Mrs. Smith, who has had two hospitalizations in the last month and declining health. The hospitalizations did not fix her end-stage heart failure. If anything, they temporized the situation, but her extreme dyspnea and other distressing symptoms will return and worsen over time.

It's time to have the talk, but how it is framed will make a difference in how a patient and their family will perceive what is being advised. It is not easy to have these conversations. In the above example, Mrs. Smith had access to a palliative care service that had broached the subject of hospice with her. Palliative care services are experts in communication. Recall that not every U.S. hospital has a palliative care service [1], and therefore many patients have not had hospice expertly presented to them. As a physician working for a hospice, you should become comfortable and competent to have these goals of care conversations and specifically address hospice care. You will need to be able to continue to speak to the hospice philosophy even after a patient has entered your hospice service. Your interdisciplinary team should also be skilled to have these conversations and complement you. Remember that you are part of an interdisciplinary care team, and the hospice care approach is one of collaboration and integration. Make sure to discuss the goals of care conversations that occurred with the patient and family at your IDG meetings. Seek input and feedback from your team members on what may have not been addressed and what can be further clarified with the patient and family.

Reference:

1. Growth of Palliative Care in U.S. Hospitals 2-22 Snapshot, New York: Centers to Advance Palliative Care, 2022 https://www.capc.org/documents/download/1031/ Accessed June 6, 2023

Further Reading:

Wittenberg E, Ferrell BR, Goldsmith J, Smith T, Ragan SL, Handzo GF. *Textbook of Palliative Care Communication*. Oxford University Press; 2016.

Back A, Arnold R, Tulsky J. *Mastering Communication with Seriously Ill Patients*. Cambridge University Press; 2009.

9.
Prognostication

The wisest have the most authority.

Plato

Physicians, in general, struggle to provide a prognosis. When we do, we are over-optimistic, especially if we have a long-established relationship with the patient. Our over-optimism may lead to late hospice referrals and delay the necessary support for patients at end-of-life [1]. The good news is that there are tools that can allow you to estimate the median life expectancy once you have determined a patient is hospice eligible. I will mention just two, the Palliative Performance Scale (PPS) and the Eastern Cooperative Oncology Group (ECOG). As you will see, there is a correlation between the number you obtain from each tool and median life expectancy.

The Palliative Performance Scale was derived from the Karnofsky Performance Scale developed in 1948 to measure performance status [2] or functionality and was later found to also be helpful as a prognostication tool for cancer patients. The Palliative Performance Scale has demonstrated that it can also be applied to other terminal, progressive diseases other than cancer. It is widely used in hospice for this reason. It measures five functional domains and is divided into 11 levels ranging from 0 to 100% [1] (Fig. 4).

%	Ambulation	Activity and Evidence of Disease	Self-Care	Intake	Level of Consciousness
100	Full	Normal Activity	Full	Normal	Full
90	Full	Normal Activity	Full	Normal	Full
80	Full	Normal Activity with Effort	Full	Normal or Reduced	Full
70	Reduced	Unable to do Normal Work	Full	Normal or Reduced	Full
60	Reduced	Unable to do hobby/housework	Occasional Assistance Necessary	Normal or Reduced	Full or Confusion
50	Mainly Sit/Lie	Unable to do any work	Considerable Assistance Required	Normal or Reduced	Full or Confusion
40	Mainly in Bed	As above	Mainly Assistance	Normal or Reduced	Full or Drowsy or Confusion
30	Totally Bed Bound	As above	Total Care	Reduced	Full or Drowsy or Confusion
20	As Above	As above	Total Care	Minimal Sips	Full or Drowsy or Confusion
10	As Above	As above	Total Care	Mouth Care Only	Drowsy or Coma
0	Death				

Figure 4. Palliative Performance Scale Tool [2].

So how do you use it? You start with the first column on the left of the tool and move across. You can move across and go down but **cannot** move across and go up. The important thing to remember is that you must go through each of the five columns.

Example:

Mr. Brown is a 78-year-old male patient with metastatic prostate cancer. He lives at home with his daughter, son-in-law, and their two teenage daughters. He has returned home after an acute hospital stay where he was treated with iv Ceftriaxone for a urinary tract infection. After his last antibiotic dose, he was discharged home by the hospitalist service. The inpatient social worker recommended a home hospice evaluation. Mr. Brown spends most of his day in bed, he is unable to do any work. He cannot self-care and requires his family to help him dress, bathe, go to the bathroom, and cut his food. His appetite has been slowly declining to where he now only eats half the food on his plate at each meal. He is confused at times.

What would you score him as on the PPS?

%	Ambulation	Activity and Evidence of Disease	Self-Care	Intake	Level of Consciousness
100	Full	Normal Activity	Full	Normal	Full
90	Full	Normal Activity	Full	Normal	Full
80	Full	Normal Activity with Effort	Full	Normal or Reduced	Full
70	Reduced	Unable to do Normal Work	Full	Normal or Reduced	Full
60	Reduced	Unable to do hobby/housework	Occasional Assistance Necessary	Normal or Reduced	Full or Confusion
50	Mainly Sit/Lie	Unable to do any work	Considerable Assistance Required	Normal or Reduced	Full or Confusion
40	Mainly in Bed	As above	Mainly Assistance	Normal or Reduced	Full or Drowsy or Confusion
30	Totally Bed Bound	As above	Total Care	Reduced	Full or Drowsy or Confusion
20	As Above	As above	Total Care	Minimal Sips	Full or Drowsy or Confusion
10	As Above	As above	Total Care	Mouth Care Only	Drowsy or Coma
0	Death				

Mr. Brown would be 30 %! You may be tempted to score him as 40 % based on the fact that his ambulation and activity and evidence of disease described in the first two columns fit nicely at 40%; however, as you move across his self-care intake and level of consciousness fit best in the 30% and not the 40%. Remember you move across AND down when appropriate, not just across. You will see why the % is important to prognostication.

Let's look at another example.

Mrs. Targot is a 68-year-old patient recently admitted to hospice with a primary diagnosis of end-stage chronic obstructive pulmonary disease(COPD). She is dyspneic at rest and wears 3 liters of oxygen continuously. You are assessing her in her home for the first time and want to provide a PPS score. She sits in a chair most of the day watching TV. She is unable to do any work. She requires assistance and is unable to ambulate without the use of a walker. She consumes approximately 75% of her meals which are of normal consistency without any concerns for aspiration. She is fully conversant and interactive.

What would you score her on the PPS?

%	Ambulation	Activity and Evidence of Disease	Self-Care	Intake	Level of Consciousness
100	Full	Normal Activity	Full	Normal	Full
90	Full	Normal Activity	Full	Normal	Full
80	Full	Normal Activity with Effort	Full	Normal or Reduced	Full
70	Reduced	Unable to do Normal Work	Full	Normal or Reduced	Full
60	Reduced	Unable to do hobby/housework	Occasional Assistance Necessary	Normal or Reduced	Full or Confusion
50	Mainly Sit/Lie	Unable to do any work	Considerable Assistance Required	Normal or Reduced	Full or Confusion
40	Mainly in Bed	As above	Mainly Assistance	Normal or Reduced	Full or Drowsy or Confusion
30	Totally Bed Bound	As above	Total Care	Reduced	Full or Drowsy or Confusion
20	As Above	As above	Total Care	Minimal Sips	Full or Drowsy or Confusion
10	As Above	As above	Total Care	Mouth Care Only	Drowsy or Coma
0	Death				

Again you may be tempted to score her as a 50% as ambulation and activity and evidence of disease fit in the first two columns fit at that level, however, as you continue your assessments, she drops in the next three columns to 40%. Her score would therefore be 40% and not 50%.

Document explicitly your findings for each column and then state that the patient's PPS corresponds to an X % based on the data. Paint the picture of decline. This would allow any other team member to understand how and why you score a patient at that particular %. PPS will change as patients decline and should be updated when a decline is noted. Once again, spell out the decline, and don't just place a number in your documentation. Your team will appreciate your thoroughness as it will make it easier for the entire team to follow the patient's decline. The percentage number alone does not help make the case for the decline.

Another tool specifically for cancer patients as their primary terminal diagnosis is the Eastern Cooperative Oncology Group (ECOG). The tool uses a 5-

point scoring system to assess performance status in cancer patients and was developed in the 1960s. It is considered a simple tool for clinical use to help assess performance status and allow oncologists to decide on chemotherapy [3]. It can as we will see also be used to help with prognostication.

Grade	ECOG
0	Fully active, able to care on all pre-disease performance without restrictions
1	Restricted in physically strenuous activity but ambulatory and able to carry our work of light or sedentary nature
2	Ambulatory and capable of self-care but unable to carry out any work activities. Up and about more than 50% of waking hours.
3	Capable of only limited self-care, confined to bed or chair more than 50% of waking hours.
4	Completely disabled. Cannot carry out any self-care. Totally confined to bed or chair
5	Death

Figure 5. ECOG tool [3].

Example:

Mr. Gee is a 79-year-old male patient with stage 4 lung cancer. He has undergone chemotherapy and also immunotherapy. He has decided to stop all disease-directed care. His oncologist has referred him to hospice. As you visit him for the first time you encounter a frail, cachectic patient who is disoriented to time sitting in a recliner watching TV. His son is present and informs you that he helps his Dad out of bed each morning and helps him sit in the recliner for most of the day. When you ask if he spends more than 50% of his day in the recliner, the son confirms that is the case.

Where would you score Mr. Gee on the ECOG?

Grade	ECOG
0	Fully active, able to care on all pre-disease performance without restrictions
1	Restricted in physically strenuous activity but ambulatory and able to carry our work of light or sedentary nature
2	Ambulatory and capable of self-care but unable to carry out any work activities. Up and about more than 50% of waking hours.
3	Capable of only limited self-care, confined to bed or chair more than 50% of waking hours.
4	Completely disabled. Cannot carry out any self-care. Totally confined to bed or chair.
5	Death

Mr. Gee would be an ECOG = 3.

Let's see another example.

Mr. Sellett is a 76-year-old male patient with metastatic colon cancer, He is undergoing chemotherapy. The patient is completely dependent on all his activities of daily living and requires maximal assistance from his elderly wife and daughter. He is bedbound and requires to be placed in a wheelchair to be transported by his wife. The patient is disoriented times two. He is evaluated by the palliative care physician at the request of his treating oncologist who speaks to the wife and daughter and recommends hospice.

Where would you score Mr. Sellett on the ECOG?

Grade	ECOG
0	Fully active, able to care on all pre-disease performance without restrictions
1	Restricted in physically strenuous activity but ambulatory and able to carry our work of light or sedentary nature
2	Ambulatory and capable of self-care but unable to carry out any work activities. Up and about more than 50% of waking hours.
3	Capable of only limited self-care, confined to bed or chair more than 50% of waking hours.
4	Completely disabled. Cannot carry out any self-care. Totally confined to bed or chair
5	Death

Mr. Sellett would be an ECOG = 4

Why would you and your hospice team want to use these tools? What do these numbers tell us? By adding these tools to your assessment of the patient, you may be able to further narrow down the prognosis beyond the initial six months at the time of hospice enrollment. We can also use these tools to help us compare a patient's cognition, functionality, and nutrition over time and help us construct a strong narrative to support continued eligibility for hospice.

Table 2. Comparison of ECOG and PPS scores and corresponding median survival in days [4].

ECOG	Median survival in days	PPS Scale	Median survival in days
0	293		
1	197	100 % to 80 %	215
2	104	70 % to 60 %	119
3	55	50 % to 40 %	49
4	25.5	30 % to 10 %	29
5	Death	0 %	Death

You can use these tools to estimate the median survival days [4]. When addressing prognosis, these are approximations, and you should carefully explain that to your patient and their families. Let's look at the examples again and tie in the median survival for each score based on the table.

Mr. Brown, our first patient with prostate cancer, has a PPS of 30%. He would, therefore, likely have a median survival of 29 days.

Mrs. Tergot, our patient with COPD, has a PPS of 40%. She would have a likely median survival of 49 days.

Mr. Gee is our patient with metastatic lung cancer. He scored a 3 on the ECOG. He would have a likely median survival of 55 days.

Mr. Sellett, our patient with metastatic colon cancer, has an ECOG score of 4. He has a likely median survival of 25.5 days.

Again, these are median survival estimates and not specific prognoses for your patient. These tools are to be used in conjunction with a detailed description of the patient's clinical course. Describe your patient's decline in regards to their functionality, cognition, and nutrition, and use these tools to help you paint the picture of a patient in the end-stage of their disease.

References

1. Warm E. Fast Fact and Concept #30 Prognostication. Palliative Care Network of Wisconsin. May 2015.

2. Baik D, Russell D, Jordan L, Dooley F, Bowles KH, Masterson Creber RM. Using the Palliative Performance Scale to Estimate Survival for Patients at the End of Life: A Systematic Review of the Literature. *J Palliat Med*. 2018;21(11):1651-1661. doi:10.1089/jpm.2018.0141

3. Azam F, Latif MF, Farooq A, et al. Performance Status Assessment by Using ECOG (Eastern Cooperative Oncology Group) Score for Cancer Patients by Oncology Healthcare Professionals. *Case Rep Oncol*. 2019;12(3):728-736. Published 2019 Sep 25. doi:10.1159/000503095

4. Jang RW, Caraiscos VB, Swami N, et al. Simple prognostic model for patients with advanced cancer based on performance status. *J Oncol Pract*. 2014;10(5):e335-e341. doi:10.1200/JOP.2014.001457 https://pubmed-ncbi-nlm-nih-gov.proxy-hs.researchport.umd.edu/25118208/

10.
The Imminent Patient

> *To be prepared is half the victory.*
> Miguel de Cervantes

Mrs. Brown is an 81-year-old patient with end-stage heart failure admitted to hospice three months ago. She was transferred to the inpatient hospice unit after she was assessed as having uncontrolled shortness of breath. You are the hospice physician and when examining the patient, you find that she is completely unresponsive, her mouth is open and her neck is hyperextended. She has livedo reticularis over her shins and her digits are blue in both hands. Her Foley tube and bag are empty and have not been voided by the RN. The family is at the bedside.

Mrs. Brown is imminent and likely has days to hours to live. The signs and symptoms listed in Table 3 when observed help you provide further prognostication information to families.

Table 3: Symptoms and signs of imminent patient [1].

Symptom/ Sign
Pulseless Radial Artery
Inability to Close Eyes
Grunting
Respiratory Mandibular Movements (Fish Gulping)
Audible secretions
Decreased Urine Output (less than 100cc in 12 hours)
Cheyne-Stokes Breathing pattern
Non-reactive pupil
Decreased response to verbal stimuli
Drooping Nasolabial Fold
Hyperextended Neck
Decreased Response to visual stimuli

The more symptoms and signs of imminence a patient may have, the higher the chance they are about to die. Patients may also have their eyes and mouths open, in addition to the other signs and symptoms listed in Table 3. Educating the family about these signs allows us to offer them a prognosis of days to hours. The psychosocial team should also prepare the family and ensure funeral arrangements are in place. As uncomfortable as this may seem, it is essential to address funeral arrangements with patients and families, and this should be discussed and reviewed for each patient during each interdisciplinary group (IDG) meeting.

You and the rest of the interdisciplinary team should have documented these signs and symptoms in your assessments and stated that you have provided the primary caregiver and family a likely prognosis of days to hours.

Let's look at another case.

Mr. Grindar is a 67-year-old male patient admitted to hospice with a primary diagnosis of end-stage renal failure a month ago. He elected to stop hemodialysis. At the time of admission, the hospice team informed his son that the median survival after stopping hospice was approximately 2 weeks. Mr. Grindar has become less responsive and is completely bedbound. He is sleeping up to 16 hours during the day. When he is awake he is confused. He started running a 100.1 fever last night. He is barely eating a teaspoon of food.

His son asks you in the follow-up visit how much time his father has?

We can further refine our prognostication of an imminent patient and provide more insight to families about the stage of imminence a patient may be at (Table 4) [2].

Table 4. Stages of Imminence [2].

	Stages of Imminence
Early	• Bedbound • Loss of interest • Loss of ability to drink/eat • Increased time sleeping • Delirium
Middle	• Obtundation with only brief periods of wakefulness
Late	• Fever- Usually from aspiration pneumonia • Irregular breathing • Apnea • Mottled extremities

If we were to take into account the median survival of an end-stage renal failure patient off hemodialysis assuming he was utterly dependent and we factor in poor cognition, nutrition, and apnea it would be reasonable to inform Mr. Grindar's son that we are looking at likely a few days to hours before his father will pass away.

Your hospice patient's imminent status should be discussed at the IDG meeting. The patient's hospice RN and the team social worker should plan to visit the patient as soon as possible. We will see when we review hospice program quality measures that their visit is an important Centers for Medicare and Medicaid (CMS) measure of quality hospice care.

References

1. Schneiderman H, Marks S. PHYSICAL EXAMINATION OF THE DYING PATIENT. *FAST FACTS AND CONCEPTS #392*. Published online January 2020.

2. Alsuhail AI, Punalvasal Duraisamy B, Alkhudhair A, Alshammary SA, AlRehaili A. The Accuracy of Imminent Death Diagnosis in a Palliative Care Setting. *Cureus*. 2020;12(8):e9503. Published 2020 Aug 1. doi:10.7759/cureus.9503

11.
Prognostication Funnel

> *A man should be upright, not be kept upright.*
>
> Marcus Aurelius

Figure 6 is a little visual aid that can help you visualize the way I approach prognostication. Where would we place any particular patient on the prognostication funnel when using all data from exams, and assessments by all IDG members, and the use of prognostications tools such as PPS, and ECOG?

We cannot be specific about how much time a patient may have remaining but we can offer families a reasonable range of time.

We can speak of the following ranges:

- Months to weeks
- Weeks to days.
- Days to hours

Start with the chronic disease trajectory the patient fits into (Fig 2).
Recall that the star is the point in the disease trajectory graph that marks the terminal phase where hospice can be offered.

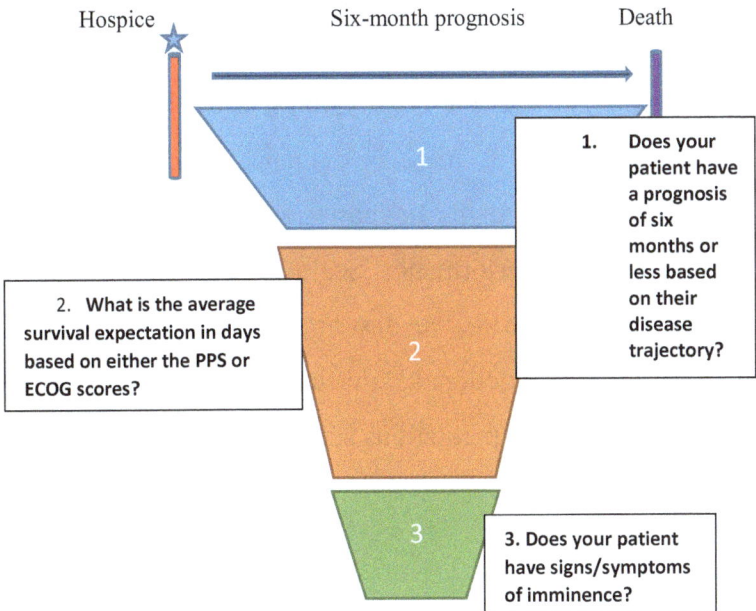

Figure 6. Prognostication funnel.

The prognostication funnel allows you to organize prognostication information and narrow the range.

Patients are eligible for hospice if they have a prognosis of six months or less of life should their terminal disease run its natural course. Consider that not every patient admitted to hospice will necessarily have a prognosis of months, especially if admitted very late when they may already be imminent. The opposite is also true.

A hospice patient may momentarily plateau and live longer than the initial six months. This is why we can re-certify patients for 60-day days after the initial six months as long as there is evidence of decline[1]. The interdisciplinary team can approximate a prognosis using the Palliative Performance Scale or ECOG for cancer patients, along with the description of the domains of impairment (functional, nutritional, and cognitive) collected through meticulous serial assessments.

Reference

1. Code of Federal Regulations Title 42 Chapter IV Subchapter B Part 418 Hospice Care. National Archives and Records Administration.https://www.ecfr.gov/current/title-42/chapter-IV/subchapter-B/part-418 Accessed June 5, 2023

12.
Code of Federal Regulations

> *There are lots of people who mistake their imagination for their memory.*
>
> Josh Billings

If you practice as a hospice physician, you must know the hospice regulations or what are known as the conditions of participation(CoPs). Hospice is codified in Title 42, Part 418 of the Code of Federal Regulations (CFR). These are the Centers for Medicare and Medicaid's regulations for hospice care in the United States. The link in the reference section will take you to Part 418 of the Code [1]. You can download and print the pdf. I highly recommend keeping the link and a copy handy as it spells out the conditions of participation. There are 8 subparts in the Code of Federal Regulations (CFR) for hospice, of which one is reserved and not completed. I am listing them here for you:

Subpart A: General Provisions and Definitions

Subpart B: Eligibility, Election, and Duration of Benefits

Subpart C: Conditions of Participation: Patient care.

Subpart D: Conditions of Participation: Organizational Environment

Subpart E : (Reserved)

Subpart F: Covered Services

Subpart G: Payment for Hospice Care

Subpart H: Coinsurance

Each subpart provides the details about the conditions of participation (CoPs), that belong to topics in that subpart. I am not going to go through each subpart but I will mention some of the essential conditions of participation you should be familiar with on day #1. They may be out of order since I am trying to group them so they make the most sense for you. Remember to review all of them and become familiar with them, especially the ones you as a physician play a key role in.

All the conditions of participation for hospice will begin with a 418, followed by a dot and then another number.

Let's jump right into Subpart B.418.20[1] states that for a patient to be eligible to elect hospice under Medicare, they must be entitled to Medicare Part A and be certified as terminally ill. Recall who is eligible for Medicare Part A as covered earlier in the guide. So for how long does a patient receive hospice? 418.21[1] clarifies that a patient receives an initial 90 days and then a subsequent 90 days (which adds up to six months). What happens if the patient outlives the initial six months? They can be recertified for an unlimited number of 60-day periods as long as they are considered terminal.

Who determines that a patient is terminal? As per 418.22[1] "For the initial 90-day period the hospice must obtain written certification statements from the medical director of the hospice OR the physician member of the hospice interdisciplinary group AND the individuals attending physician if the individual has an attending physician ….". You need **two** physicians to certify a patient initially to allow them to access their first 90-day period. For the second 90-day period and subsequent periods, you only need one physician to certify the patient. This is a task usually completed by the hospice physician. That would be you.

What are we doing when completing a certification? We are informing CMS that in our clinical judgment, the patient is at a terminal stage of their qualifying disease and is eligible to access hospice. When we re-certify them, we attest that the patient is still declining and continues to be eligible for hospice.

What happens if the patient is not Medicare Part A eligible? Patients may become terminal before reaching 65, in which case they will likely be enrolled in Medicaid, or they may have private insurance. Usually, both Medicaid and private insurance will follow Medicare regulations. There may be particular differences for patients covered by private insurance carriers, and you should become familiar with any differences if your patient is covered by a private insurance carrier. You will sometimes be called upon to interact with private insurance companies who may need help understanding the specific mechanics of hospice. The good news is that you should be able to discuss and educate on how hospice works after reading this guide.

Let me give you an example:

Mrs. Green is a 62-year-old female recently admitted to hospice with a terminal diagnosis of COPD. She is on 2 liters of oxygen via nasal cannula for disabling dyspnea at rest. She is 5 out of 6 activities of daily living dependent and scored as having a Palliative Performance Scale score of 50%. She becomes very anxious and calls 911. EMS services, unaware the patient is on hospice, transport an anxious and extremely short-of-breath patient to the nearest ED. Your hospice program is informed the patient has been hospitalized. The hospice

RN visits the patient. The patient is agreeable to continuing on hospice. The case is discussed with the hospital's case manager. She is placed on a hospice contract bed overnight and will be discharged home to continue home hospice the next day.

Mrs. Green is not eligible for Medicare Part A and is still covered by private insurance. You are asked to discuss the case with the Utilization Medical Director of the insurance company, as her hospitalization coverage was declined. The Utilization Medical Director informs you that Mrs. Greene, at very best, could be considered observation status and does not qualify for inpatient. You must explain that the patient is in hospice, and observation vs. inpatient for hospitalization does not apply in hospice. You will likely need to educate the Utilization Medical Director on the 4 levels of hospice care and that Mrs. Green met general inpatient level(GIP) for an uncontrolled symptom that could not be reasonably managed in the home setting. Read on. It will make sense as we review the four levels of hospice.

What Needs to be Documented?

42 CFR 418.22(b)[1] states that the certification of a patient's terminal condition is based on the physician's or medical director's **clinical judgment** of the normal course of the individual's illness. I want to clarify a couple of things here for you.

1. You may not be the official medical director of your program, however, it clearly states physician or medical director, so if you are the hospice physician directly taking care of the patient this does refer to you. Your clinical judgment.
2. There are Medicare Administrative Contractors (MAC) that oversee the administration of hospices in the U.S. They each have a specific geography they cover. Each one has a list of local coverage

determinations for specific disease states (dementia, cancer, congestive heart failure, COPD, etc.).Understand that these local coverage determinations are guidelines that should help you paint the picture as you are documenting why your patient is eligible to access their hospice benefit. The ultimate authority here is not the MAC's local coverage determinations but your clinical judgment! Not everything is going to have all the right check marks or fit nicely into a box. Remember to refer to the chronic disease graphs. Where is your patient on the graph? What are their limitations as far as domains of impairment? Describe them and don't be afraid to state that in your clinical judgment, the patient has a prognosis of 6 months or less should the terminal illness run its normal course.

What needs to be stated in hospice documentation?

As per 418.22 (b)(1)[1] "The certification must specify that the individual's prognosis is for a life expectancy of 6 months or less if the terminal illness runs its normal course".

This statement should be included in all your documentation. As a physician you should construct a narrative, indicating the clinical finding that supports a life expectancy of six months.

Let's look at two examples of documentation for the same patient:

Example # 1.

Mr. Moss is being admitted to hospice after having been hospitalized for gangrene of his left foot. He was hypotensive. Palliative medicine was consulted and hospice was recommended. He has a prognosis of six months or less.

Example # 2.

Mr. Moss is a 68-year-old male patient with end-stage systolic heart failure, CKD stage 4, brittle uncontrolled diabetes mellitus who was hospitalized for gangrene of his left foot. During his hospitalization patient was determined to have delirium. The patient is not able to follow commands or engage in conversation. He is poorly interactive with his environment. The patient is bedbound, not able to do any activities of daily living, and requires total care. His food and liquid intake is reduced to only 25% of previously consumed meals consisting of a puree consistency diet. He is considered at high risk for aspiration due to the presence of cough and pocketing when eating. He is confused. He is scored as having a palliative performance scale score of 30%. As per previously reviewed records patient weighed 170 pounds 3 months ago. Today his weight is 143 pounds indicating that he has lost 27 pounds in the last 3 months.

Based on the above data and personal exam of the patient, it is my clinical judgment that Mr. Moss has a prognosis of six months or less should his terminal disease run its normal course. He is eligible for initiation of hospice with a primary diagnosis of end-stage systolic heart failure.

Same patient, but as you can see, example # 2 paints a more accurate picture of a patient in their terminal phase. Example # 1 needs to make a stronger case for hospice eligibility. You want to be specific and explicit when constructing your narrative to support your initial certification and re-certifications. Your narrative should be **distinct and appropriate for each patient** reflecting the decline expected to occur over time. 42 CFR 418.22(b)(3)(iv)[1] specifically addresses not to copy and paste your narrative. Copy and paste and generic statements are easy to spot.

After the initial 180 days or the first two 90 certification periods, a face–to–face encounter MUST occur with the patient. A thorough assessment including a complete physical exam is to be performed at every face-to-face encounter. This visit can be performed by an advanced nurse practitioner (that is employed by hospice (It cannot be an independent nurse practitioner) or any other physician working for the hospice. Per 42 CFR 418.22(b)(4)[1] in the face-to-face documentation the nurse practitioner (APRN) or certifying physician must state:

1) Face-to-face encounters occurred with the patient.
2) Date of the encounter
3) Clinical findings were provided to the certifying physician for use in determining continued eligibility for hospice.

When constructing your re-certification, it is good practice if you did not perform the face–to–face exam to reference who performed, it, on what day, and that you are using the exam as part of your determination for continued eligibility for hospice. Be meticulous with your documentation. Remember that you are dealing with a federal entitlement program.

The rules about the timing of completing documentation!

You should remember The first specific number in the CFR is for the Notice of Election (NOE). Patients or their representatives must file a notice of election within five **(5)** calendar days after the effective date of the election statement. The NOE informs CMS that an eligible hospice patient has enrolled in end-of-life care. In essence, this allows services under Medicare Part A to flip into hospice care. Hospices will facilitate paperwork for patients and families.

A comprehensive assessment needs to be completed upon admission. Per 42 CFR 418.54(b)[1], an initial comprehensive assessment identifying the patient's, physical, psychosocial, emotional, and spiritual needs must be completed within five **(5)** calendar days from admission.

42 CFR 418.54(d)[1] speaks to the ongoing comprehensive assessments that must be accomplished by

the hospice interdisciplinary group as frequently as the patient requires but no less frequently than every fifteen (**15**) days. What it is addressing is that a hospice patient's holistic interdisciplinary care must be discussed at a very minimum every fifteen (**15**) days with the entire IDG. There is no other part of our healthcare system in the U.S. where a plan of care for a patient is reviewed this frequently. I highlight this critical distinction about hospice care when educating primary caregivers and families. Families may not realize that every person who comes into contact with the patient will then meet to discuss the care provided to the patient as a team. Based on the discussion at the IDG meeting, the plan of care should be documented in the patient's chart.

As per 42 CFR 418.22(a)(3)(ii)[1], you can complete a certification up to fifteen (**15**) days before the effective date of election. This would never really be an issue as certification usually occurs after the patient has elected and been enrolled in hospice. Interestingly enough, this is also true for any of the re-certifications. You could therefore construct a certification narrative up to 15 days before a patient enrolls in hospice. For a patient in hospice who you have concluded will continue to be eligible, you can complete the re-certification narrative, but, make sure that this is done no more than 15 calendar days before the next subsequent benefit period begins.

Example:

Mr. Frome admitted to hospice with a primary diagnosis of end-stage cerebral atherosclerosis, will enter his 3rd certification period on June 25. You could complete the re-certification from June 11 onward. What you cannot do is complete the re-certification on June 5. Think of it this way: CMS gives you a 15-day head start to complete the paperwork, so you don't have to do it on the spot and have enough time to do a great job.

What about the face-to-face visit timing?

As for 42 CFR 418.22(a)(4)(i)[1] states it can be and should be completed before the start of the third benefit period and for any subsequent benefit period; however, it cannot be completed any sooner than thirty (**30**) days before the benefit period begins. CMS is giving you thirty (**30**) days to complete the face-to-face so it can be used for re-certification.

Let's see an example to clarify this condition of participation. If we go back to Mr. Frome's case, we could have the hospice APRN complete a face-to-face on May 26th for you to use in your re-certification documentation. What you cannot do is use a face-to-face that is older than 30 days before the beginning of the certification period. What if the APRN has an excellent face-to-face note before the 30 days? It's a no-go! Either they complete a new exam, or you must go out and have a face-to-face while ensuring it is within the 30 days before the re-certification is due.

Remember to sign and date all certification and re-certification and document the certification period 42 CFR 418.22(b)(5)[1]. This is a no-brainer, but you might be surprised that something may be missed. Attention to detail! Always! You are dealing with CMS.

Reference

1. Code of Federal Regulations Title 42 Chapter IV Subchapter B Part 418 Hospice Care. National Archives and Records Administration.https://www.ecfr.gov/current/title-42/chapter-IV/subchapter-B/part-418 Accessed June 5, 2023

13.

Medicare Administrative Contractor

Nothing comes merely by thinking about it.

John Wanamaker

Just look at the Code of Federal Regulations and all the regulations for hospice care. Imagine if a clinic or a hospital practice was regulated in the Code of Federal Regulation as it is for hospice care. CMS does not directly oversee hospice but relies on the Medicare Administrative Contractors to do so.

"A Medicare Administrative Contractor (MAC) is a private health care insurer that has been awarded a geographic jurisdiction to process Medicare Part A and Part B (A/B) medical claims or Durable Medical

Equipment (DME) claims for Medicare Fee-For-Service (FFS) beneficiaries [1]." Yes, another layer of complexity to our healthcare system in the U.S. CMS relies on a network of MACs to oversee and administer the Medicare FFS program and the healthcare providers who serve Medicare patients. MACs perform many activities including:

1. Process Medicare FFS claims
2. Make and account for Medicare FFS payments
3. Enroll providers in the Medicare FFS program
4. Handle provider reimbursement services and audit institutional provider cost reports
5. Handle redetermination requests (1st stage appeals process)
6. Respond to provider inquiries
7. Educate providers about Medicare FFS billing requirements
8. **Establish local coverage determinations (LCDs)**
9. Review medical records for selected claims
10. Coordinate with CMS and other FFS contractors

I will call your attention to #8. These private insurance contractors establish the local coverage determinations (LCDs) for hospice care. There may be variations in local coverage determinations according to each MAC. There are four MACs for Hospice in the United States [1].

Image 2. Medicare Administrative Contractor for Hospice in the U.S.[1]

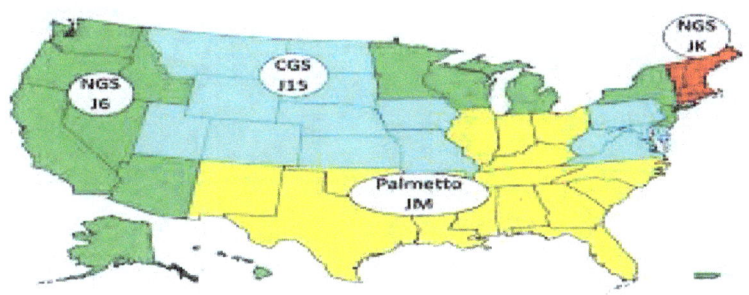

A terminal patient may not neatly fit into a MAC's local coverage determinations. Unfortunately, some out there may interpret them as rules and that a terminal patient must meet these local coverage determinations to be hospice eligible. The local coverage determinations help you construct the narrative to show that a patient is eligible for their hospice benefit. They should not prevent you from determining hospice eligibility. Recall from the Code of Federal Regulations that your **clinical judgment** as a physician is the ultimate final word for hospice eligibility. Remember that it is the terminal prognosis, not the diagnosis, and only physicians can offer a prognosis to patients, not private insurance companies or the government. Hopefully, you understand the importance of why I covered prognostication in an earlier chapter.

Here is an example:

Mrs. Goodwin is an 82-year-old female patient with advanced COPD. She has been hospitalized for acute shortness of breath and started on an antibiotic regimen. She has poor compliance with her oxygen which she is supposed to use continuously. She has been hospitalized twice in the last year, including the most recent hospitalization for acute respiratory failure. You are asked to assess the patient. She is dependent on dressing, transferring, and toileting, and needs 1-person assistance to complete these tasks. She can cut her food. Her daughter informs you her food intake has decreased, and she has lost at least 10 lbs. in the last two months. She is in a hospital gown, so you are not able to comment if her garments are loose-fitting. Before hospitalization, the patient was able to ambulate with the use of a walker. You assess her as having a PPS of 40%. You do think based on your assessment that she would be hospice eligible and discuss your finding with the hospitalist who agrees and is willing to be the second certifying physician.

Let's see what the local coverage determination from the Palmetto MAC says about a patient with Pulmonary Disease [2].

There are three things the MAC lists as helping you support terminal prognosis:

    1. Severe lung disease which can be supported by
        a. Disabling dyspnea at rest

      b. Progression of end-stage pulmonary disease as evidenced by increasing ER visits or hospitalizations.
2. Hypoxia at rest on room air, evidenced by a pO2 of less than 55 mmHg or O2 saturation of less than 88%.
3. Other factors to support the terminal diagnosis:
      a. Right heart failure
      b. Unintentional progressive weight loss of greater than 10% in the preceding six months.
      c. Resting tachycardia of more than 100 beats per minute.

We know Mrs. Goodwin has had at least two recent hospitalizations. She has not had an arterial blood gas (ABG) during this hospital stay (It was ordered by the

ED physicians, but the patient refused), so we cannot comment on pO2 of less than 55 mmHg. You do find that her O2 was 85% when she first arrived at the ED. There are no records to specify the presence of cor pulmonale (alteration in structure and function of the right ventricle) and no recent ECHO reports for the patient to review. You know she has lost weight, but you are not certain if it is more than 10% in the preceding six months, but can take a good guess by looking at the patient and speaking with the family. Her heart rate has not been above 100 in all the records. Can you certify her for hospice? Is it reasonable to consider she has a prognosis of six months or less?

Mrs. Goodwin is declining. She is dependent on 3 of 6 ADLs and has had weight loss with a noted decrease in food intake. You have assessed her as having a PPS of 40%, which would give you a median survival of less than six months. She is not exactly fitting the local coverage determinations for end-stage lung disease. She will, however, meet the condition of participation – your clinical judgment! Use what you can from the LCD to construct the case, make sure you are meeting all the necessary conditions of participation, and finish strong by clearly stating that the patient is eligible based on your clinical judgment.

The local coverage determinations are guidelines and should help you make the most robust case possible, but you may not always find they will fit exactly for each patient. Find your MAC and look at their local coverage determinations. There may be differences from one MAC to another. Remember these are private companies contracted by CMS.

I want you to be clear on the difference between Conditions of Participation and Local Coverage Determinations. We abide by the Conditions of Participation we take into consideration the Local Coverage Determinations. Table 5 will help you visualize the differences between the two.

Table 5. Difference between CoPs and LCDs.

Organization	Term	Compliance	Source
U.S. Government	Conditions of Participation	*Mandatory*	Code of Federal Regulations
Medicare Administrative Contractors (Private companies)	Local Coverage Determinations	Guidelines to help you with eligibility.	Can obtain specific MAC LCDs (Quick flips)

Your hospice company may also have internal policies and best practices you should become familiar with.

Hospice is a federal entitlement program, overseen by private companies (MACs) on behalf of the federal government, and provided by private hospice agencies, whether they be for profit or not for profit. As you can see, you and your team have several layers of bureaucracy above you and your team. Can you see how this would be confusing and daunting to patients and their families?

There is a series of books that cover local coverage determinations according to which MAC covers your area in the U.S. The Quick Flip hospice books can be bought on Amazon.com. They are a helpful resource, and I suggest picking up a copy.

References

1. Who are the MACs. CMS.gov. https://www.cms.gov/medicare/medicare-contracting/medicare-administrative-contractors/who-are-the-macs. Accessed July 3, 2023

2. A Guide for Hospice Medical Directors. Hospice Quickflips. The Corridor Group 2017.

14.

Patients Stopping Hospice Care

Men are never so good or so bad as their opinions.

James Mackintosh

Patients may revoke from hospice at any time and for any reason as explained in 42 CFR 418.28(a)[1]. Patients will, as per 418.24[1], return to their prior Medicare coverage if they revoke from hospice. Here is something to think about. We use prognosis to establish hospice eligibility, but there is no consideration for prognosis if a patient returns to Medicare Part A. If a patient was carefully considered for hospice due to a terminal condition with an expected prognosis of six months or less if their disease ran its natural course, then returning to Medicare Part A and all its services would make little sense. This is a weak point in the regulations. As per the conditions of Participation, two physicians must certify the patient as terminally ill. When a patient revokes hospice, there is no need for direct physician involvement. A patient returns to the previous care level in Medicare just before they began hospice. All the support provided by the hospice interdisciplinary team, coverage of medications for symptom management, and equipment go away.

I stress how important it is to clarify expectations and goals when discussing hospice enrollment and of all subsequent hospice team interactions with the patient and family. Does the patient understand they are terminal?

Let me share an example:

Mr. Jimenez is an 88-year-old with stage 4 lung cancer. He was admitted to hospice 2 weeks ago. Since admission to hospice, he has noticed his symptoms, namely his dyspnea improved. He has decided after speaking to his family that he wants to return to his oncologist who has offered to proceed with more chemotherapy.

As a hospice physician, I would recommend understanding the patient's rationale for discontinuing hospice. What are they hoping for? Diplomatically and compassionately discuss the patient's expectations in seeking treatment or intervention outside of hospice. Are there other issues outside the physical domain not being addressed? Remember that you have a whole interdisciplinary team that can and should address any psychosocial, emotional, or spiritual needs the patient may have. Does the situation merit a visit by the entire team to the patient's home?

Our job as hospice physicians is to make sure we have done our best to explain their disease trajectory and where they are on that trajectory based on all we know about the patient. Disease-directed treatment and interventions are not likely to change where the patient is on their disease trajectory, and most importantly, these treatments and interventions will not improve their quality of life.

Reference

1. Code of Federal Regulations Title 42 Chapter IV Subchapter B Part 418 Hospice Care. National Archives and Records Administration.https://www.ecfr.gov/current/title-42/chapter-IV/subchapter-B/part-418 Accessed June 5, 2023

15.

Discharge from Hospice

As we advance in life, we learn the limits of our abilities.

James Anthony Froude

As per 42 CFR 418.26(a), [1] hospice can discharge a patient for three reasons:

1. The patient moves out of the service area or decides to transfer to another hospice.

2. The hospice determines the patient is no longer terminally ill.

3. The patient or others in the patient's home have disruptive or abusive behavior or are uncooperative and cause serious disruption to the provision of hospice care.

Let's look at some examples.

Scenario # 1:

Mrs. Greene is a 75-year-old female patient with a primary hospice diagnosis of COPD. She was admitted to your hospice 2 months ago. She lives at home with her daughter Mary, who has to relocate to another city for work reasons. Mary has discussed the situation with her sister Susan who has agreed to have Mrs. Greene come live with her. Susan lives in Arizona. Mrs. Greene and Mary presently live in Texas.

Your hospice does not have a program in Arizona. Your social worker investigates the closest hospice program to Mrs. Greene's new residence, calls ahead, and provides Mary and Susan the information to establish follow-up and enrollment with the new hospice once she arrives in Arizona. She will be discharged from your hospice since she is leaving your service area. Upon admission to the new hospice, she will continue with her present certification period.

The second scenario is when a patient is determined no longer to be terminally ill. Your hospice likely has a review process for these cases. Before pulling the trigger to discharge, review the case meticulously and discuss the situation with the IDG. Make sure everyone taking care of the patient has a voice and can express questions, doubts, or concerns. The decision to discharge a patient should not be taken lightly and should be a team decision based on a consensus that the patient is no longer believed to be terminal.

Scenario # 2:

Mr. Joseph is a 66-year-old male patient admitted to hospice with a primary diagnosis of end-stage diastolic heart failure. He was admitted after an acute hospitalization for CHF exacerbation. The family had noted the decline in his ability to complete his activities of daily living. His appetite had been decreasing over three months before hospice admission. He was reported to be confused and withdrawn at the time of admission to the hospital. His PPS was 40% at the time of admission.

A year has gone by, and the patient is alert, awake, and oriented times three. He can ambulate with the use of a walker and without assistance. There have been no falls. He has gained 10 lbs. and is eating 100 % of his meals which are regular consistency, with no concerns for aspiration. Since admission, he has not had any infections or required escalation of services to either continuous care or GIP level. As the case is reviewed with the IDG, it is concluded that there is indeed a struggle on the part of the entire IDG to find objective evidence of decline.

It is concluded that at this time, the patient is chronic and not terminal and will therefore be discharged from hospice according to 42 CFR 418.26(a)(2)[1].

Ensure that the case is carefully and thoroughly reviewed and that a visit for the patient has been recently completed to corroborate that there is no objective evidence of decline and that the patient is being discharged based on the best information and in good faith. The patient and family should be made aware ahead of time that the IDG will review hospice eligibility and may proceed to discharge the patient. It is good practice to have ongoing discussions with the patient and family about the lack of objective findings of decline if this is what is observed. It is also important to educate patients and families about the Medicare Hospice Benefit regulations regarding discharge if a patient is not found to have evidence of decline. Discharging a patient from hospice should never be abrupt and a surprise to the patient and family.

Scenario #3:

Mrs. Gonzales is an 80-year-old female patient with a primary hospice diagnosis of cerebral atherosclerosis. She was determined to be completely dependent on all her activities of daily living on admission. Her palliative performance scale score was determined to be 30%. She had been hospitalized for a urinary tract infection and treated with antibiotics before being referred to hospice. The hospitalist presented artificial nutrition and hydration as an option to the family, and the family did not wish to consider PEG placement.

Mrs. Gonzales has been under your hospice service for two years. Her case is being reviewed due to the prolonged length of stay. Her case is discussed at the IDG. She remains completely dependent on all her ADLs.

She has noticeable muscle wasting in all four extremities and her garments are loose-fitting. She is non-verbal and she has recently completed a course of antibiotics. She has been more dyspneic and her oxygen requirements have gone up. You have ordered her oxygen to be increased from 2 liters to 3 liters continuously by nasal cannula and she is also on q 6 hourly albuterol nebulization.

Mrs. Gonzales has outlived her six-month prognosis! However, to the best of your IDGs assessments, she continued to show objective evidence of decline. Should you proceed to discharge? No! There may have been a point in the last two years where Mrs. Gonzales was not showing decline and could have been discharged. This is why paying attention to prognostication on admission is essential, and we should use all the tools we have to make the best decision at each encounter point with the patient. What we should not do is discharge a patient who is declining because they have outlived their initial six-month prognosis. Remember that you can continue to recertify for unlimited 60-day periods as long as you can support terminality and continued decline.

Scenario #4:

Mrs. Jones is a 48-year-old female admitted to hospice a month ago with a primary diagnosis of ovarian cancer. She was placed on Methadone for pain control. At the IDG, the patient's RN informs you that the patient uses oxycodone and fentanyl patches she had stocked up before her admission to hospice. She also has requested an early refill on her breakthrough morphine. Both the social worker and chaplain inform you that the patient has denied them entrance to her home and told them she does not want to meet with them and is not interested in their services. They have made several attempts to meet with her. You have visited Mrs. Jones and discussed the appropriate use of the prescribed opioid regimen and have informed her that you will not be able to continue to provide care if she does not abide by the agreed plan of care you have discussed. She has agreed on several occasions to follow the plan of care, however, the RN continues to bring to the team's attention that she is taking non-hospice-prescribed opioids and is not following the hospice plan of care.

What to do?

42 CFR 418.26(a)(3)[1] gives you the guidance for discharge for cause:

1. Advise the patient that discharge for cause is being considered.
2. Ensure the team has made the necessary effort to resolve the problem caused by the behavior.
3. Make sure that the proposed discharge is not due to the

patient's use of necessary hospice services

4. DOCUMENT! DOCUMENT! DOCUMENT! The effort made by the team and make sure it is in the medical record.

You would need an extraordinary case such as this one to discharge a terminal patient. Make sure the team is engaged and that the decision to move forward with discharge is based on an interdisciplinary assessment, and that every possible reasonable effort has been made to resolve the situation, but it is not possible to safely continue to provide hospice care. A tough case such as this one can pop up. Discharges for cause are rare and should be exceptional cases in hospice care.

As per 42 CFR 418.26(b)[1], for a patient to be discharged from hospice, there must be a WRITTEN order from the physician. You should document that you have provided a safe discharge plan, including educating and counseling patients, caregivers, and the family. As per 42 CFR 418.26(d)[1] you have established a clinical follow-up visit with the patient's primary care physician or arranged for a primary care physician to follow the patient after discharge if they do not have one. Do not forget that the hospice must file a notice of termination of election within five(**5**) calendar days after discharge as per 42 CFR 418.26(e) [1].

Reference

1. Code of Federal Regulations Title 42 Chapter IV Subchapter B Part 418 Hospice Care. National Archives and Records Administration.https://www.ecfr.gov/current/title-42/chapter-IV/subchapter-B/part-418 Accessed June 5, 2023

16.

The Hospice Team

Our lives are universally shortened by our ignorance.

Herbert Spencer

I want to once more clarify as I did in the introduction that the official language in the Code of Federal Regulations speaks of interdisciplinary group. A group is a set of people considered together because they have something in common. For example, an IDG has in common that they work for the same hospice. Each group member may have independent goals, accountability, and success [1]. A team the other hand is a group of people interdependent and working towards a common goal. The team shares those common goals and holds each other accountable to achieve those goals [1]. Our goal in hospice is to provide the best possible end-of-life care. I work in a team and not in a group. Be aware that we use interdisciplinary group (IDG) and not interdisciplinary team in our hospice documentation as that is the language used in the Code of Federal Regulations. I do not think that they considered the difference between group and team when the CFR was drafted. Perhaps they will eventually reconsider. Until then just remember which one to use when you are documenting. In spirit, we are part of a hospice team. On paper, we are part of a hospice group.

A little then on the hospice interdisciplinary group.

As per 42 CFR 418.56(a)(1)[2], "The hospice must designate an interdisciplinary group or groups composed of individuals who work together to meet the physical, medical, psychosocial, emotional, and spiritual needs of the hospice patients and families facing terminal illness and bereavement. Interdisciplinary group members must provide the care and services offered by the hospice, and the group, in its entirety, must supervise the care and services". The interdisciplinary group must include, but is not limited to, individuals who are qualified and competent to practice in the following professional roles:

Core Services **THAT MUST BE PROVIDED**

- A doctor of medicine or osteopathy (who is an employee or under contract with the hospice).
- A registered nurse.
- A social worker.
- A pastoral or other counselor (Bereavement, Dietary, Spiritual).

A hospice physician MUST work as part of a team and demonstrate that the care provided is interdisciplinary. That is the essence of what hospice is all about.

As per 418.102 [2], a physician can serve as a hospice physician or a medical director, and the only requirement is to be a doctor of medicine or osteopathy. Unlike a clinic practice or hospital setting, there are no residency, fellowship, or board certification requirements to serve as a hospice physician.

Non-Core Services.

These services may be provided if available and if reasonable in addressing quality of life.

- PT/OT/ Speech pathologist

There is a misunderstanding that therapy services cannot be provided for hospice patients. If they are considered to be beneficial and improve quality of life, they can be requested. As a physician, you should clarify with the patient and caregiver that if available to your hospice, these services have a limited scope and are not being provided to restore functionality. The decline will continue to occur. If that were not the case, then the patient would not be eligible for hospice care.

- Hospice aides

Hospice aides work under the direct supervision of the patient's hospice nurse. The work on providing personal care, assisting RNs, assisting with ambulation and exercises, and can assist with administering medications that would usually be self-administered 42 CFR 418.76(g)(2)[2]

- Volunteer services

As per CFR 418.78(e)[2], **5** percent of the total patient care hours should be provided by volunteer services. This was designed to maintain a sense of community on which the hospice philosophy was founded. Volunteers provide many essential support services for patients and families. They are also part of the hospice interdisciplinary team.

Reference

1. Asana. Group vs. Team: What's the Difference? • Asana. Asana. Published October 14, 2021. https://asana.com/resources/group-vs-team

2. Code of Federal Regulations Title 42 Chapter IV Subchapter B Part 418 Hospice Care. National Archives and Records Administration.https://www.ecfr.gov/current/title-42/chapter-IV/subchapter-B/part-418 Accessed June 5, 2023

17.
Hospice Medications

Nothing endures but change.

Heraclitus

A common myth about hospice is that electing hospice means stopping all the patient's medications. Patients and families may offer resistance to hospice because they are under the impression that their medications will be discontinued. Therefore, it would help ease patients and families to clarify this issue on day #1. As per 42 CFR 418.54(c)(6)[1]: a comprehensive review of the patient's present medication regimen needs to be undertaken. The effectiveness of any drug in current use should be reviewed, as well as its side effects. If the patient has been identified as having difficulty swallowing, then the pill burden should be addressed. We help decrease the risk of aspiration by agreeing with the patient and family to eliminate medications with low or no benefit. Potential drug interactions with medication you may need to add to address symptoms should be reviewed and discussed with the patient and their family. This is an opportunity to eliminate duplicate medications that may address the same symptom. Any drug requiring laboratory monitoring should be identified. If these drugs are to be continued who will be ordering and following laboratory monitoring should be clarified. Before stopping any medications, the risk/benefit of any chronic medication should be discussed with the patient and with their surrogate. A rationale should be clearly explained as to why a medication's risks or burdens outweigh its potential benefits. This is all part of the initial goals of care discussion you and the hospice team should have with patients and their families.

What if the patient wishes to continue on a medication unrelated to their terminal diagnosis? Hospice patients are still covered by Medicare Part D and can continue to receive the medication if their primary care physician or specialist continues to prescribe it. This is why medication-relatedness must be discussed and addressed on admission to hospice.

Let's look at an example:

Mr. Wiley is a 69-year-old patient admitted to hospice with a primary diagnosis of end-stage heart failure. He also has intermittent A-Fib, and his cardiologist had placed him on Warfarin which was later changed to Apixaban for stroke prevention.

Is Apixaban covered by hospice? No

Why? Apixaban is prescribed to reduce the patient's risk of embolic stroke. It is a preventive measure, not an intervention to palliate a symptom at end-of-life. The risk of a possible embolic stroke is measured in years not months (CHA2DS2 VASc or CHADS2 scores) [2]. A patient enrolled in hospice has an expected prognosis of six months or less.

Does it make sense to continue medication to reduce stroke risk if the prognosis is less than six months?

Deprescribing Apixaban and the rationale should be discussed with the patient and their family. They may not wish to stop it, and their primary care physician or specialist may want to continue it. As they have a prescribing physician, the medication will be covered under Medicare Part D. Patients will need to pay the co-pay[2] for medications covered under Medicare Part D.

There is a great flow chart from the NHPCO that you can reference to help you navigate what may be related or unrelated [3]. Sometimes there may be a clear clinical justification to cover a medicine that may initially seem like it is not related when it may indeed be. This is where your expertise as a hospice physician will be needed and valued.

Certain medications are ALWAYS related to hospice and need to be documented as such.

Let's look at an example:

Mrs. Logly is a 79-year-old female patient admitted to hospice with a primary diagnosis of end-stage COPD. She is on MS Contin (long-acting morphine)15 mg po q 12 hours for chronic non-malignant pain. She is on Senna (Sennakot) 8.6 mg po q night for constipation prevention. She has been nauseated and she was recently prescribed Zofran (ondansetron) 4 mg po q 8 hours prn.

Which of the above medications would be related to her hospice care?

Trick question! All of them!

The morphine, Sennakot, and Ondansetron are all hospice's responsibility to cover.

Any medication prescribed for a hospice patient to treat:

- Pain
- Nausea
- Constipation
- Anxiety

is assumed by Medicare to be ALWAYS covered by hospice [4]. Documentation should reflect that any medications used to address any of the above 4 categories of conditions are related and are therefore being covered by hospice.

References

1. Code of Federal Regulations Title 42 Chapter IV Subchapter B Part 418 Hospice Care. National Archives and Records Administration. https://www.ecfr.gov/current/title-42/chapter-IV/subchapter-B/part-418 Accessed June 5, 2023

2. Gažová A, Leddy JJ, Rexová M, Hlivák P, Hatala R, Kyselovič J. Predictive value of CHA2DS2-VASc scores regarding the risk of stroke and all-cause mortality in patients with atrial fibrillation (CONSORT compliant). *Medicine (Baltimore)*. 2019;98(31):e16560. doi:10.1097/MD.0000000000016560

3. Determination of Hospice Medication Coverage. NHPCO. April 2020 Version 1.0

4. Drug Coverage under hospice. Medicare Rights Medicare Interactive. https://www.medicareinteractive.org/get-answers/medicare-covered-services/hospice/drug-coverage-under-hospice. Accessed July 7, 2023

18.

The Four Levels of Hospice Care

It's not what you look at that matters, it's what you see.

Henry David Thoreau

1.) **Routine home care:** Hospice was intended to be provided in the comfort of a patient's home. Hospice services are available 24/7 but are not present in the home 24/7. Be careful how this concept is communicated, as patients and families will struggle with the perceived amount of needed support and may feel that they are not receiving enough. They may misunderstand that someone from hospice will be in the home, primarily assisting with ADLs. A family may misunderstand, for example, the role of the health aide who, among other things, helps with bathing. They may misinterpret this resource as being available in the patient's home for the entire day. The patient may need 24 hours round the clock supervision. Ensure to explicitly address that hospice will not provide this level of supervision. Good practice would be to clarify what is being provided and, if a gap is identified, be able to provide a list of community resources that can supplement the care needs of the patient. The reality is that primary caregivers, mostly close family members, are likely providing anywhere between 40 to 60 hours of care per week [2]. The Code of Federal Regulations does not address primary caregivers or their needed qualifications. These caregivers are more likely to suffer from depression, anxiety, or poor physical health. Your hospice IDG should also address the reality of the caregivers, physical, emotional, and financial well-being[2]. Can the primary caregiver realistically provide the needed care and supervision? Routine home care is not as simple as it may seem on paper and requires a lot of engagement and support by the entire IDG, including the hospice physician.

2.) **Continuous home care:** To be provided when there is an uncontrolled symptom in the home. Care is to be provided by an RN for at least 8 hours out of 24 hours, beginning and ending at midnight. This care should only be provided for a crisis due to an uncontrolled symptom. The patient should return to routine home care as soon as the symptom is resolved.

What services count towards continuous care hours? Only direct care that is provided predominantly by nursing (RN or LPN) employed by hospice, and any care provided by hospice-employed nurse practitioners and hospice aides. social worker's and chaplain's hours are not counted as part of continuous care hours.

We should not confuse reimbursement rules with expected team support. Yes, the social worker and chaplain are not included in billable services, but it would be hard to make a case that their presence would not be required during a crisis. As we will see later under quality reporting, a social worker's visit to an imminent patient measures hospice care quality. Would it be reasonable to consider a hospice patient in a crisis to possibly progress toward an imminent state or already be there? I would say yes. So, if the social worker were not to go, and the patient was imminent and expired your hospice quality measures will be negatively impacted.

When is continuous care not appropriate?

- No acute pain or symptom management needs even if the patient is imminent.
- Caregiver breakdown with no pain or symptom management needs.
- Using continuous care for respite care
- For safety concerns (patient falling or wondering) if there are no skilled interventions.
- As an alternative to paid caregivers or placement in another setting.

Continuous care can be provided in a private residence, assisted living facility(ALF), or skilled nursing facility(SNF) [4]. I want to stress here that it would also be important to provide a physician visit if symptoms are not resolving with the ordered interventions you have directed the nurse to provide. The nurse should be communicating with you on the progress of the patient.

3.) Respite care: To be provided to patients when the patient's primary caregivers need to take a break from caregiving or need to take a trip and require the patient to be supervised. Respite care cannot be used if there is no identified caregiver. Suppose a patient resides in a nursing facility that provides 24/7 care. In that case, respite-level care cannot be provided as the patient should receive adequate supervision from the nursing facility staff. And, of course, if there is no apparent reason for respite care. Respite care is provided for 5 days. On day six, the hospice will be compensated at the routine home level of care. You should also know that as per 42 CFR 418.302(f)[1], the total number of respite days is included as part of the calculation for inpatient care where a hospice may not exceed more than 20 percent of inpatient days for their beneficiaries in 12 months (See below) [3].

4.) General Inpatient Care: To be provided for symptom management that cannot be feasibly managed in the home setting GIP documentation should support the level of service. You should be able to describe what is specifically being provided and support why this care cannot be provided at a different level of hospice [5]. What was attempted for the patient before escalating care to GIP? What are the specific symptoms being addressed, what interventions are being provided, and what are the results of the interventions?

Condition of participation 42 CFR 418.108(d)[1] is a little peculiar, and you should know what it states.
"The total number of inpatient days used by Medicare beneficiaries who elected hospice coverage in a 12-month period in a particular hospice **may not exceed 20 percent of the total number of hospice days consumed in total by this group of beneficiaries**." If you recall from the second chapter, we have a hospital-centric healthcare system in the U.S.

I mention this because patients and families may struggle once in an inpatient hospice unit with being discharged back to routine home hospice care. Despite the interdisciplinary team approach, there may be gaps in care the primary caregiver and family may feel they cannot meet. The transition back home may not be as seamless as it should be. It is imperative to start discharge planning from admission to a general inpatient care level as well as work with your interdisciplinary team on a safe transition back to the routine home level of care.

Example:

Mr. Julos is an 82-year-old male patient with metastatic prostate cancer to bones. He was on oral Methadone at home but was assessed as having a pain crisis and no longer responding to the pain regimen. His pain regimen was adjusted, but the patient was still in crisis, and it was decided that the best course of action was to admit him to the hospice inpatient unit for initiation and titration of a patient-controlled analgesia pump (PCA) with frequent physician and nursing monitoring.

Once Mr. Julos's pain is controlled and there are no further interventions requiring a GIP level of care, Mr. Julos should transition back to a routine home hospice level.

What if the caregivers object to having him return home? Complex psychosocial situations arise all the time in hospice. Remember our dependency on hospitals and inpatient care in the U.S. Again, you must rely upon and work collaboratively with the rest of the IDG to resolve the situation. You cannot, however, continue to bill Medicare at the GIP level of care if the symptoms are resolved. The patient will need to be transitioned to an alternative level of care even if remaining physically in the location where the GIP level of care was being provided. Hospice will bill Medicare routine home hospice level. Families will likely be made responsible for room and board. As a physician, you must order the level of care change. It is your responsibility!

References

1. Code of Federal Regulations Title 42 Chapter IV Subchapter B Part 418 Hospice Care. National Archives and Records Administration. https://www.ecfr.gov/current/title-42/chapter-IV/subchapter-B/part-418 Accessed June 5, 2023

2. Agarwal A, Alshakhs S, Luth E, et al. Caregiver Challenges Seen From the Perspective of Certified Home Hospice Medical Directors. *Am J Hosp Palliat Care*. 2022;39(9):1023-1028. doi:10.1177/10499091211056323

3. Managing Medicare Hospice Respite Care. National Hospice and Palliative Care Organization. Compliance Tools and Resources. Revised July 2021. https://www.nhpco.org/wp-content/uploads/Respite_Tip_sheet.pdf Accessed July 10, 2023

4. Continuous Home Care in the Medicare Hospice Benefit. Respite Care. National Hospice and Palliative Care Organization. Compliance Tools and Resources. Revised March 2021 https://www.nhpco.org/wp-content/uploads/CHC_Compliance_guide.pdf. Accessed July 10, 2023

5. Hospice General Inpatient (GIP) Level of Care Frequently Asked Questions. National Hospice and Palliative Care Organization. Compliance Tools and Resources. July 2021 https://www.nhpco.org/wp-content/uploads/GIP_FAQs.pdf Accessed July 10, 2023

19.

Hospice Funding

> *Education is the art of making man ethical.*
> Georg Wilhelm Friedrich Hegel

There are many articles out there that speak of hospice as a multibillion-dollar industry. Remember that hospice is part of Medicare Part A. Before falling into the trap of thinking we are spending excessive money on hospice, consider the following. Hospice providers, whether they are labeled for-profit or not-for-profit hospice only receive less than 1/10 of the total funding for Medicare Part A.

Table 6. Congressional Budget Office Medicare Spending[1].

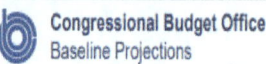
Congressional Budget Office
Baseline Projections

Medicare

By Fiscal Year, Billions of Dollars

	Actual, 2021	2022	2023	2024	2025	2026	2027	2028
BUDGET INFORMATION								
Medicare Totals								
Mandatory Outlays[a]	868	983	1,019	1,034	1,165	1,262	1,360	1,541
Discretionary Outlays	8	7	8	9	9	10	10	10
Gross Outlays	875	991	1,027	1,043	1,174	1,272	1,370	1,552
Total Offsetting Receipts[b]	-180	-216	-170	-181	-198	-216	-234	-253
Net Outlays (Gross outlays minus receipts)	695	775	857	862	976	1,056	1,137	1,299
Net Mandatory Outlays	688	768	848	853	967	1,047	1,127	1,289
Components of Mandatory Outlays								
Benefits								
Part A	354	388	404	410	454	481	508	562
Part B	413	475	494	503	570	616	669	765
Part D[c]	98	119	119	118	138	163	181	212
Total Benefits	865	981	1,016	1,031	1,162	1,260	1,358	1,539
Mandatory Administration[d]	2	2	2	3	3	2	2	2
Total Mandatory Outlays	868	983	1,019	1,034	1,165	1,262	1,360	1,541
Components of Benefits								
Hospital Inpatient Services	147	145	146	150	155	159	165	170
Skilled Nursing Facilities	29	28	27	28	28	28	28	29
Physician Fee Schedule	66	72	73	70	69	70	71	73
Hospital Outpatient Services	60	64	66	70	75	81	88	96
Home Health Agencies	17	17	17	17	18	18	19	19
Group Plans (Includes Medicare Advantage)	340	427	460	463	557	611	668	794
Part D[e]	98	119	119	118	138	163	181	212
Low-income subsidy (Non-add)	34	43	42	41	48	46	47	55
Other services[f]	108	109	108	115	122	130	138	146
Total Benefits	865	981	1,016	1,031	1,162	1,260	1,358	1,539
Components of Offsetting Receipts								
Part A Premiums	-4	-5	-5	-5	-5	-5	-5	-6
Part B Premiums[g]	-114	-131	-133	-142	-156	-170	-185	-201
Part D Premiums[h]	-6	-6	-6	-6	-7	-8	-8	-9
Part D Payments by States	-12	-12	-15	-16	-17	-19	-20	-22
Payments Recovered from Providers[i]	-45	-63	-12	-13	-13	-14	-15	-17
Total	-180	-216	-170	-181	-198	-216	-234	-253

Take a look at Table 6. As a point of illustration, I have highlighted the total spending for Medicare Part A in 2021. A total of 354 billion dollars was spent just on Medicare Part A [1]. What was the spending for hospice care in 2021?

23.1 billion [2].

Let's do a little math here. 23.1 billion dollars out of a total of 354 billion dollars represent 6.52% of the total Medicare Part A budget.

Next time you read one of those sensational headlines about the multibillion-dollar hospice industry keep the above percentage in mind. Hospice is not such a money maker, is it? Ask yourself where the lion's share of Medicare Part A is spent. Recall that we spend ¼ of the total Medicare budget on beneficiaries in their final year of life. We are spending money on acute hospitalizations, interventions, and procedures that will not impact the patient's prognosis. I wonder why there are not more stories about this topic in the media?

The table will hopefully help you calculate the percentage of the total hospice spend compared to the total spend for Medicare Part A over the next several years [1]. As you can see, we will keep spending more and more money on Medicare Part A and, of course, more on hospice, but something tells me the actual percentage spent on hospice will not dramatically change.

Now let's look at how CMS spends money on hospice to provide end-of-life care. So, what is the Hospice Wage Index? Every year CMS provides a figure known as the Hospice Wage Index that indicates the amount of money CMS will spend for each Medicare beneficiary enrolled in hospice. Hospice is a capitated system, meaning there is no further funding for hospice care once the maximum Hospice Wage Index is spent for each beneficiary for that year. The figure will continue to increase year to year, and the amount paid out varies depending on where the hospice is located in the U.S. Would it not be interesting if our payroll tax collection to cover Medicare Part A varied by where we live in the U.S.? They don't! I am implying that a beneficiary who has paid into the Medicare Part A fund should receive the same amount of money for their hospice benefit irrespective of where they live. You should know that the Hospice Wage Index amount is and will be tied to penalties and metrics for each hospice and that CMS is still fine-tuning how they will roll out metrics and changes. The variation in what is paid out would make sense if it was solely based on the quality of the hospice care that is provided and not on where a beneficiary or their hospice is located. I stress this point to make you aware that funding is impacted by a patient's location. As a federal entitlement program a patient should receive the same level of care irrespective of where they live in the U.S. Is that possible is there is variation in the funding?

You will face important financial considerations when moving patients from one of the four levels of hospice to the other.

So let's look at the **proposed** Fiscal Year 2024 Hospice Wage Index. The Cap amount, meaning the amount CMS will pay for each hospice patient annually, is maxed at $33,396.55 [2]. Seem like a lot of money?

Compare that to the average cost of one single hospitalization for a Medicare beneficiary at $13,600 [3]. Add a procedure or intervention, and that figure is likely to be much higher. Also, consider that a patient with multiple chronic medical problems and declining health is likely to access the hospital several times as the symptom burden increases and worsens as their health declines. If we make a cost comparison providing holistic, interdisciplinary care through hospice makes more sense financially. Having patients at the end of life return to the acute care setting of a hospital and seek care that can be provided at home does not make clinical sense. It is also unlikely that end-of-life patients will receive coordinated psychosocial, emotional, and spiritual care in the hospital. Hospice is about providing holistic care and support to patients and their families while being good stewards of our healthcare resources, which are not unlimited. As you can see, context is everything. You can read more on the Hospice Wage Index under 42 CFR 418.306(b) [5].

CMS will compensate hospice organizations on a per diem basis, and depending on the level of hospice service intensity, the per diem rate will vary. Consider that this per diem includes all needed core and non-core services, any medications related to the terminal diagnosis, and needed durable home equipment.

As a way to exemplify this, I am including the **likely** 2024 reimbursement rates for each level of service. Keep in mind that these rates change and you will need to stay on top of what the figures are from year to year.

Table 7. Proposed payment rates for hospice level of services in 2024 [3].

Level of Hospice Service	Payment rate
• Routine Home Care Days (1 -60)	$ 217.74
• Routine Home Care Days (+61)	$ 171.86
• Continuous Home Care (Full 24 hours)	$ 1.561.63
• Respite Care	$ 506.38
• General Inpatient Care	$ 1.142,20

Hospice is intended to be provided primarily in the home setting. Most of a patient's care is expected to be at a routine home care level. In 2024 for the initial 61 days, CMS will pay a per diem rate of $217.74. After day 61, the rate goes down to 171.86. Remember, this is for everything provided by hospice for the care of the patient.

Let's look at some examples of the implications of transferring to a higher level of care or using respite care.

Mr. Jones is a 69-year-old patient admitted to hospice 4 months ago with a primary diagnosis of end-stage COPD. He is on 2 liters of oxygen, ipratropium-albuterol nebs every 6 prn, and immediate release morphine 5 mg q 6 hours prn. His family is planning to attend a wedding out of state. They remember the initial conversation at the time of admission about respite care and would like hospice to care for their father while they are out of town attending the wedding.

Of course, your hospice should be able to honor this request; however, it is vital to inform the family that we can provide respite for 5 days. Look at the difference in per diem reimbursement between routine home care and respite care. Respite care costs more!

Let's review another scenario.

Mrs. Thomas is a 77-year-old patient with metastatic breast cancer. She has been in hospice for 4 months. Your hospice RN calls to inform you that she is noticeably short of breath. The RN informs you that she has crackles at the bases and new pitting edema at the ankle. She is on 2 liters of oxygen on a needed basis at home. You ask the RN to elevate the head of the bed, place the patient on 2 liters of oxygen continuously, and start Furosemide 40 mg po once a day. You ordered her to be started on continuous home care, which means the patient will have 24-hour RN supervision, and plan to visit her tomorrow.

Take a look at the per diem reimbursement rate for continuous care. Yes, $1,561.53 per day of service; compare that to the routine home care rate. **Continuous care is the most expensive level of hospice care.** There should be clear documentation of the symptom, the interventions provided, and how they impact the symptom. Continuous care should be discontinued once the symptom is controlled, and the patient should return to the routine home level of care. Recall that hospice is a capitated system. If the patient does not require this level of service because there are no uncontrolled symptoms, you would be billing CMS for an unnecessary level of hospice care. As the hospice physician, you are responsible to enter the level of care change.

Let's look at the same case with an escalation in the level of care.

Mrs. Thomas remains on continuous care for three days but is not improving with the interventions that are being provided. It is decided to send her to one of the hospice's inpatient units. Her daughter Julia is her proxy and agrees to provide iv opioids to help mitigate her respiratory distress. Mrs. Thomas was transferred to the IPU and started on a Morphine drip.

General inpatient care is compensated at $ 1.142.20 per day. It is the next most expensive level of hospice. Surprised? Most people are as they would think that general inpatient is the most expensive level. Once again, symptom burden and interventions provided to address the symptom and outcome should be documented to support the GIP level of service. Once the symptom is resolved, the patient should return to routine home care. Not doing so places you at risk if your hospice is audited. In the best-case scenario, your hospice must issue a refund to CMS. Worst case scenario? You are a licensed physician dealing with the U.S. government and billing for a level of service that is not justified! This can be potentially viewed as Medicare fraud.

My intent here was to show you that there are financial and legal implications with the use of the four levels of hospice service. I also hope you can contrast the overall cost of end-of-life and what the cost would be without hospice as a patient may continue to seek hospitalizations even though they are at the end of life.

References

1. Congressional Budget Office Baseline Projections May 2022.https://www.cbo.gov/system/files/2022-05/51302-2022-05-medicare.pdf Accessed June 26, 2023

2. End-of-Life Care and Hospice Costs. Debt.org. June 16, 2023, https://www.debt.org/medical/hospice-costs/ Accessed June 22, 2023

3. NHPCO Analysis of the FY 2024 Hospice Wage Index and Quality Reporting Proposed Rule. https://www.nhpco.org/regulatory-and-quality/regulatory/billing-reimbursement/ Accessed June 22, 2023

4. Charaba C. Infographic: How much does a hospital stay cost? Published January 12, 2023BC. https://www.peoplekeep.com/blog/infographic-how-much-does-a-hospital-stay-cost Accessed June 22, 2023

5. Code of Federal Regulations Title 42 Chapter IV Subchapter B Part 418 Hospice Care. National Archives and Records Administration.https://www.ecfr.gov/current/title-42/chapter-IV/subchapter-B/part-418 Accessed June 5, 2023

20.

The Hospice Patient and the ED

> *Wisdom denotes the pursuing of the best ends by the best means.*
>
> Francis Hutcheson

In the U.S., patients have been conditioned to use the emergency department for any perceived emergency. Hospice patients experiencing distress from uncontrolled symptoms will call 911 if their care needs are perceived as not being addressed on time.

Let's take a look at an example:

Mrs. Lucien is an 81-year-old female patient with end-stage cerebral atherosclerosis with vascular dementia. She has suffered several falls over the last couple of months. She can no longer ambulate with the aid of a walker and has been completely bedbound for the last two weeks. She was referred to hospice by her primary care physician after discussion and agreement with her eldest daughter, whom the patient had designated as a healthcare surrogate for medical decisions. This morning her youngest daughter visited her mother and found her more confused. The hospice team provided education about hospice philosophy and prognosis on admission and at every point of interaction with the family. The patient's daughter called the hospice RN, who informed the daughter that she would be arriving to visit the patient within the hour. The daughter, in a panic, calls 911. Mrs. Lucien is taken to the closest ED. In the ED, she undergoes a battery of tests, including chest X-ray, CBC, BMP, Troponin, and D-dimer. Her troponin and D-Dimer returned abnormally high, and she was sent for a CT Chest PE protocol which is reported positive for clots in both lung vasculatures. She was started on a heparin drip and admitted to the hospital.

    This is a common scenario we face in hospice. I have to wonder if the education provided only included the patient's eldest daughter, who had agreed to hospice. Was her youngest daughter present during the initial hospice discussion, and if so, what did she understand? Were concepts about end-of-life clearly explained? Was a disease trajectory graph used to help the family visualize where the patient was on her disease journey? Were hospice care concepts and philosophy reinforced at all further encounters by the hospice team?

The ED may not know that this is a hospice patient. Believe it or not, this also happens. This may have been a detail that may have escaped the EMS service. Because the family did not mention it, and there was no visible documentation to show that she was a hospice patient. We need to find ways to improve the identification of hospice patients so that EDs can first clarify goals of care before initiating work-ups which will likely not change the prognosis or impact the patient's quality of life [1].

As a hospice physician, you may be asked to determine if the diagnosis used for the hospital admission is RELATED or UNRELATED. Here is where there may be confusion, as there may be a misunderstanding that a condition or diagnosis is only related if it is tied to the patient's primary hospice diagnosis.

In the case of Mrs. Lucien, you may think that a pulmonary embolism is not related to her primary hospice diagnosis of cerebral atherosclerosis. Wrong! I am going to point you to her disease trajectory graph. She is in hospice. Did we consider her PPS score? Right, she is a terminally ill patient. If not, she would not be in hospice. Is it reasonable to think that a bedbound patient can develop a blood clot? Yes. Can a pulmonary embolism be fatal? You bet. Can it contribute to shortening the six-month prognosis? Absolutely. Is it related? YES.

Recall that a hospice patient or their healthcare proxy can revoke hospice services at any time for any reason as per the conditions of participation. First, you will want to clarify with the patient's family if they wish for Mrs. Lucien to remain in hospice and continue with symptom management. If they answer yes, you can see if the hospital and your hospice have an agreement to provide a bed for general inpatient hospice (contracted hospital bed) or move the patient to one of your hospice inpatient units.

What about the heparin drip? This is where you will need to be a great hospice physician and once again help the family focus on the goals of care. Will the heparin drip extend the patient's life? What are the burdens of therapy? Do the benefits of anticoagulation outweigh the risks? Mrs. Lucien would need to transition eventually to oral anticoagulants. These things should be discussed transparently and compassionately with the family.

I will leave you the link to the National Hospice and Palliative Care flow chart for Related Conditions in reference [1]. I suggest you print it and have it handy to reference and share it with the rest of your hospice team.

Reference

1. NHPCO Relatedness Process Flow_Revised Version 2.0 2020vFinal. National Hospice and Palliative Care Organization. https://www.nhpco.org/regulatory-and-quality/regulatory/determining-terminal-prognosis/attachment/nhpco-relatedness-process-flow_revised-version-2-0-2020vfinal/ Accessed June 15, 2023.

21.
Primary Care and Other Physicians

> *A prudent question is one-half of wisdom.*
>
> Francis Bacon

Patients need to elect their attending as per 418.52 (c)(4) [1]. The hospice physician will serve in that role if they still need one. Per the Code of Federal Regulations, the hospice physician should coordinate care needs with the patient's primary care. This is an important concept for you to speak about, as primary care physicians in the community may misperceive that they are losing patients to hospice. The Hospice Medicare Benefit was designed to maintain the primary care physician and incorporate them into the interdisciplinary care team. Ideally, if the primary physician remains engaged in the care of a hospice patient, there are two physicians providing care. The hospice physician is responsible for all the care related to the terminal condition, while the primary care physician can provide care for all non-terminal conditions.

When primary care physicians are unavailable irrespective of the patient's needs, the hospice physician must address any clinical needs. As per 42 CFR 418.64[1], "If the attending physician is unavailable, the medical director, contracted physician, and/or hospice physician employee is responsible for meeting the medical needs of the patient." That means also addressing non-hospice conditions when needed.
Let me give you a specific example to clarify this last point.

Mrs. Smith, who was admitted to hospice with a primary diagnosis of end-stage systolic heart failure, also has diabetes. Her primary care physician is still managing her diabetes and treating her with a Lantus and Novolog insulin regimen. It is Friday night and the patient's daughter calls the hospice. She is concerned as the patient's Accu check is reading 400 mg/dl. The daughter has tried calling the PCPs office but has not received a callback.

As the hospice physician, you must manage the hyperglycemia and adjust the insulin regimen even though it is not part of the hospice care plan. You are also obligated to contact the primary physician, inform the primary care of what adjustments you made, and provide a safe handoff and agreement on ongoing clinical management by the primary care physician.

Primary care physicians and other physicians can continue caring for hospice patients. That is because patients do not lose Medicare Part B. However, it should be understood that physicians outside of hospice will bill Medicare Part B and that patients will be responsible for any co-pays as this is outside of hospice. This is clearly stated in condition of participation 418.402[1], which speaks about the liability of the Medicare deductibles and coinsurance payments and the difference between the reasonable and actual charge on unassigned claims on other covered services that are not considered hospice care. Patients and families may not be clear about this and you and your team may need to address this.

Examples of services not considered hospice care include:

- Services furnished before or after a hospice election period
- Services of the individual's attending physician, if the attending physician is not an employee of or working under an arrangement with the hospice
- Medicare services are received for the treatment of an illness or injury not related to the individual's terminal condition.

How to use billing modifiers

There are two billing modifiers for Medicare claims you should become familiar with to help educate community physicians. These are modifiers non-hospice physicians may use when rendering services to hospice patients.

GW Modifier

Service unrelated to the patient's terminal condition[2]

This modifier should be used when a service is rendered to a patient enrolled in a hospice and the service is unrelated to the patient's terminal condition.

Mrs. Smith's primary care physician would use this modifier when submitting a claim for the treatment of her diabetes as this is not a hospice diagnosis.

GV Modifier

Attending physician not employed or is paid under an arrangement by the patient's hospice provider[2]

The attending physician should use this modifier when the services are related to the patient's terminal condition or are paid under an arrangement by the patient's hospice provider. Also, this modifier must be submitted when a service meets the following conditions, regardless of the type of provider:

- The service was rendered to a patient enrolled in a hospice.
- The service was provided by a physician or non-physician practitioner identified as the patient's attending physician at the time of that patient's enrollment in the hospice program.

This would be the case when a hospice provider refers a patient to an outside provider. An example would be if Mrs. Smith was determined to be severely depressed by the hospice interdisciplinary team, and a decision was made to refer her to a psychiatrist for expert consultation. The Hospice would likely pay the psychiatrist but needs to add this modifier to the Medicare claim.

A patient and their family may decide to visit a physician or seek a service outside of the hospice plan of care without informing or discussing it with the hospice. They will as mentioned be responsible for the Medicare copay.

Not so simple, is it? Another reason why hospice care is complex.

References

1. Code of Federal Regulations Title 42 Chapter IV Subchapter B Part 418 Hospice Care. National Archives and Records Administration.https://www.ecfr.gov/current/title-42/chapter-IV/subchapter-B/part-418 Accessed June 5, 2023

2. Jitendra MS CPC When to use Hospice GV and GW modifier February 7, 2020 https://www.americanmedicalcoding.com/use-hospice-modifiers-gv-gw/ Accessed June 22, 2023

22.

Advice about Pain Management

Men are disturbed not by things, but by the view which they take of them.

Epictetus

42 CRF 418.52[1] speaks of patients' rights, and it is essential to highlight section c. **"Patients are to receive effective pain management and symptom control from the hospice for conditions related to their terminal disease.**" Patients should be educated about the scope of services that hospice will provide and the specific limitations of those services. This includes their pain and symptom management plan. Patients can refuse care or treatment, which is more likely to occur if they do not understand why a treatment is being provided.

Uncontrolled pain can interfere with sleep patterns, appetite, and energy levels, leading to fatigue, weight loss or gain, and a weakened immune system. Uncontrolled pain can also lead to increased anxiety, depression, and inability to cope. Patients and families need to be involved in developing their hospice plan of care, including pain management. It is crucial to explain the intervention to build trust in the team and the hospice plan of care.

A systemic review article by Shipton found that the average time spent learning about pain management in U.S. schools was 11 hours [1]. I call upon my fellow hospice physicians to consider the importance of actualizing and improving primary and secondary palliative care knowledge and skills. Going into pain and symptom management is well beyond the scope of this guide, and there are many excellent resources to consult. I will recommend some awesome resources I use anytime I have a question. I do want to give you an example here to illustrate why you must brush up on pain management to avoid dangerous pitfalls. As a hospice physician, you will also need to be equally skillful in other symptoms that appear at end-of-life.

Our goal in hospice is to provide high-quality end-of-life palliative care to our hospice patients. To do just that we need to practice evidence-based medicine and not intuitive medicine. It is important to understand certain nuances and be aware of them when formulating pain and symptom management interventions.

I am going to use Fentanyl patches as an example.

When considering using any opioid medication you should know the difference between opioid naïve and opioid-tolerant [3].

Any patient who has been on:
- 60 mg of oral Morphine daily
- 30 mg of oral Oxycodone daily
- 8 mg of Hydromorphone daily

For over one week is considered an opioid-tolerant patient!

Any other patient not meeting the above threshold is considered opioid-naïve!!!!

When it comes to the use of Fentanyl patches you should know that:

FENTANYL PATCHES SHOULD NEVER BE PLACED ON AN OPIOID NAÏVE patient!!!! Read again!

It may be tempting to think that a patch is a convenient way to address pain in a hospice patient. Perhaps you concluded that because they have dysphagia a patch is the best option. Or perhaps the primary caregiver is giving the team a hard time due to anxiety about having to administer opioids to their family member. Before writing the script did you assess if the patient is opioid naïve or tolerant? Is the patient's pain considered acute or chronic?

It may also be tempting to think that a 12 mcg transdermal patch should solve the problem, after all, it is the lowest TDF strength (You should know that the dose is 12.5 mcg and not 12 mcg. The FDA approved it as a bridge between doses and not as a starting dose). You would be surprised at how many hospice patients have a patch slapped on with the illusion that their pain is adequately addressed. The set it and forget it method doesn't work! Don't do it!

A 12 mcg transdermal patch is not a small dose. Next time you are about to use a 12 mcg transdermal fentanyl patch; you will need to ask yourself if you would alternatively be comfortable starting the patient on 30-to 67mg. oral morphine equivalents/day?

No! Too much? Exactly! Then you should not be using a 12 mcg transdermal patch. When considering a fentanyl patch, be aware of the oral morphine equivalents because you may be surprised that you are prescribing a high dose of an opioid that can cause harm. We want to have effective pain management, not dangerous pain management.

Is your patient in acute pain? Is a Fentanyl patch the right choice? No! Remember, we do not use Fentanyl patches for acute pain. Let's say you ignore all of the above and decide to go ahead with a Fentanyl patch, you should keep in mind that it will take at least 24-36 hours for C max (drug concentration) to be achieved. While the patch takes effect, the patient will likely still have uncontrolled pain. If the patient becomes obtunded, removing the patch is not enough as it will take almost a day for the fentanyl to be cleared [3].

What about breakthrough pain? A fentanyl patch by itself will not be enough to control pain in case of breakthrough or incident pain. You should also be providing an opioid breakthrough regimen in case your patient has an acute exacerbation of pain.

Is the patient cachectic? Not eating, losing weight? Fentanyl patches need adipose tissue to work properly [3]. (See illustration in the article on how fentanyl works as a depot in adipose tissue) [2]. Our cachectic end-of-life patients are not ideal candidates for transdermal fentanyl patches!

Does the patient have renal failure? Ah good, fentanyl is safe in renal failure patients, however, there is a better option. Methadone! Please read Dr. McPherson's white paper on methadone listed in reference [4].

Summary:

- Fentanyl patches should never be used in opioid-naïve patients! You should know if your patient is opioid naïve or tolerant, it is good medicine AND the lawyers can easily identify this when they review records.

- If you decide to use a transdermal fentanyl patch keep in mind the amount of morphine milligram equivalents, you just slapped on. It may be a very high dose and not what you intended. Remember to check your equivalency. Do the math! Our patients' pain control depends on it.

- Cachectic patients? Fentanyl is a poor choice! Where is the depot going to form?

- The patient is in renal failure and you need to give something effective? Methadone, Methadone, Methadone!

A little too much or too over your head? Good! Again I intend to call attention that you will need to be careful when using any pharmacological intervention, especially when prescribing opioids. You need to make use of references and often. As a hospice physician, you must provide effective pain and symptom management. Most importantly it has to be safe pain and symptom management.

It is crucial not only to identify a symptom but to provide an intervention and then monitor the outcome of the intervention provided. Figure 7. shows you how you should think of symptom management, monitoring, and documentation.

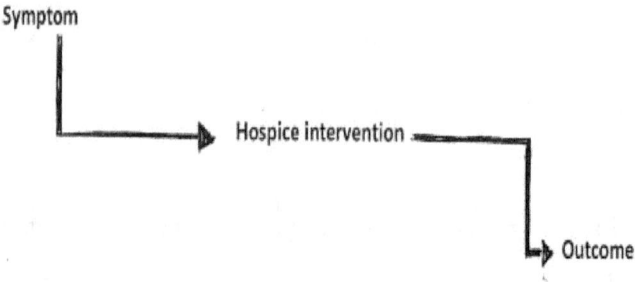

Figure 7. Symptom, hospice intervention, outcome flow diagram for pain.

Example:

Symptom: Patient complains of a 6/10 dull pain located over the left shoulder, constant, non-radiating, aggravated by moving the shoulder, alleviated by resting and avoiding moving the shoulder. The pain is impacting his appetite, which has decreased, and he has been unable to sleep comfortably due to the pain waking him up at night.

Intervention: The patient is opioid naïve and was started on Methadone 2.5mg sublingually q 12 hours with morphine sulfate 5 mg sublingually q 4 hours prn for breakthrough pain. A laxative regimen of Senna 8.6 mg po bid was added to prevent opioid-induced constipation.

Outcome: The patient reports 48 hours after starting the pain intervention that pain is 4/10 on average. He reports improved appetite and sleep. No constipation was reported.

You can be an ok hospice physician or a great hospice physician. The choice is yours and depends on your attention to detail. Your hospice should have a pharmacist. Speak with them. You share the same goal of providing safe and effective pain and symptom management to your patients.

As mentioned, it would be well beyond the scope of this guide to list all the symptoms you will encounter in hospice care. I will point you to the Fast Facts Palliative Care Network of Wisconsin database. You will find concise and well-written short hospice and palliative skills papers to help guide and validate your decision-making and provide the most effective symptom management to your patients [5]. This amazing database is also available as an app that can be downloaded on your iPhone or iPad for quick and easy access.

Here is a list of excellent references you should keep at hand to help you with pain and symptom management. Start building your reference library!

References

1. Shipton EE, Bate F, Garrick R, Steketee C, Shipton EA, Visser EJ. Systematic Review of Pain Medicine Content, Teaching, and Assessment in Medical School Curricula Internationally. *Pain Ther.* 2018;7(2):139-161. doi:10.1007/s40122-018-0103-z

2. Nelson L, Schwaner R. Transdermal fentanyl: pharmacology and toxicology. *J Med Toxicol.* 2009;5(4):230-241. doi:10.1007/BF03178274

3. Mary Lynn McPherson. *Demystifying Opioid Conversion Calculations.* ASHP; 2018

4. McPherson ML, Walker KA, Davis MP, et al. Safe and Appropriate Use of Methadone in Hospice and Palliative Care: Expert Consensus White Paper. *J Pain Symptom Manage.* 2019;57(3):635-645.e4. doi:10.1016/j.jpainsymman.2018.12.001

5. Fast Facts - Palliative Care Network of Wisconsin. Palliative Care Network of Wisconsin. Published 2019. https://www.mypcnow.org/fast-facts/

Further Reading

1. Mary Lynn Mcpherson. *Demystifying Opioid Conversion Calculations*. ASHP; 2018. YOU NEED TO HAVE THIS BOOK!

2. Berger A, O'Neill JF. *Principles and Practice of Palliative Care and Support Oncology*. Lippincott Williams &

3. Wilkins; 2021. *Essential Notes in Pain Medicine*. Oxford Univ Press; 2022.

4. Bridget Mccrate Protus, Kimbrel JM, Grauer PA. *Palliative Care Consultant : A Reference Guide for Palliative Care : Guidelines for Effective Management of Symptoms*. Hospiscript Services; 2015.

5. *Oxford Textbook of Palliative Medicine*. Oxford Univ Press; 2021.

6. *Textbook of Palliative Medicine and Supportive Care*. Crc Press; 2020.

23.

The Agitated Hospice Patient

> *A wise man proportions his belief to evidence.*
>
> David Hume

I am explicitly addressing this since this is, in my experience, the issue that families find most confusing and can lead to misunderstandings. Families may have certain expectations about a patient regaining aspects of their cognition, which are impossible due to inevitable disease progression.

Example:

Mr. Rand is an 82-year-old male patient admitted to hospice with a primary diagnosis of cerebral atherosclerosis and vascular dementia due to long-standing essential hypertension. He has progressively been confused and is now combative. The hospice RN calls you, the hospice physician, for guidance on what to do. She asks if we can start the patient on benzodiazepines to help "calm" the patient down.

You should know that benzodiazepines may worsen the agitation, cause excessive sedation and place the patient at risk for increased falls. I often see Benzodiazepines being provided without a clear rationale. They may have a place in a plan of care, but there should be a rationale reason for their use. Equally vital as you consider your interventions is to think of non-pharmacological interventions first and pharmacological interventions second.

Agitation is the third most common symptom in dementia patients after depression and apathy. It can range between 30 to 50% in patients with dementia [1]. What is essential to keep in mind is that agitation is associated with increased use of higher levels of care, increased medications, and higher mortality.

A patient with dementia may be depressed. They can also develop delirium. Table 8 hopefully helps distinguish between the three. It is not always easy or that simple to do so.

Table 8. Differentiating features between Delirium, Dementia and Depression [2].

Features	Delirium	Dementia	Depression
Onset	Acute (hours to days)	Insidious (Months to Years)	Acute of Insidious
Course	Fluctuating	Progressive	May be Chronic
Duration	Hours to days	Months to Years	Months to Years
Consciousness	Altered	Usually clear	Clear
Attention	Impaired	Normal except in severe Dementia	May be decreased
Psychomotor changes	Increased or decreased	Often Normal	May be slowed in severe cases
Reversibility	Yes	Irreversible and progressive	Usually
Present on admission		Yes or No	Yes or No

Patients with dementia are more vulnerable to delirium. Delirium may also occur in hospice patients with chronic progressive terminal diseases other than dementia. Keep in mind that hospitalizations are a known trigger for agitation. Be on the lookout for any recent hospitalization in a patient with an abrupt change in cognition. I recommend using a screening tool for delirium, such as the 4A, since it can be easily used by all the interdisciplinary team [3].

You should be able to describe the level of agitation and objectively score it. One handy tool is the Pittsburgh Agitation Scale (PAS) [4]. The PAS has four behavior groups; aberrant vocalization, motor agitation, aggressiveness, and resisting care. Each group has a scale rating the intensity of each behavior ranging from 0 to 4. A maximum of 16 points can be assigned to any patient. I recommend describing clearly what you are seeing and scoring the agitation with a tool such as the Pittsburgh Agitation Scale so that you have an objective measure and comparison to see if your interventions are effective. If you do not know where you are starting how will you know where you end up?

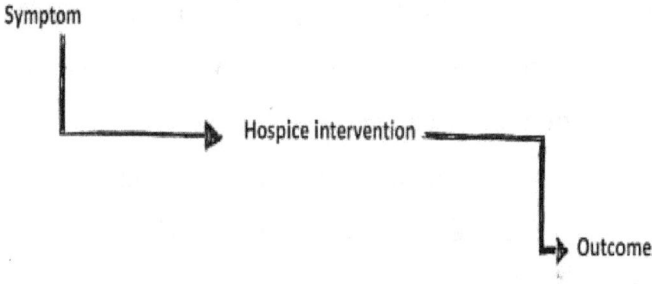

Figure 8. Symptom, hospice intervention, outcome flow diagram for agitation.

Be careful about what is being prescribed. Asides from benzodiazepines which should not be used lightly, the next common class of used medications for agitation are antipsychotics. Make sure to read up on pharmacology, especially on the side effects! Be ready to discuss these with your team and, most importantly, be able to explain them to the patient's family. Always educate the primary caregiver on why agitation is occurring. Explain your interventions and explain what we hope to achieve with the interventions. Did the primary caregiver verbalize understanding of your conversation? Good, then document it (Figure 8)! You want to make sure that your entire team is aware that the plan was discussed, and you want to go back to what was discussed and update and change the plan knowing what the initial conversations entailed. Am I being too cautious here? Look for yourself at 42 CFR 418.52(c)(8)[5], which states that patients and families receive information about the scope of services that the hospice will provide and specific limitations on those services.

Again, please build your hospice reference library and resources to learn how to effectively and safely manage symptoms at end-of-life.

References

1. Carrarini C, Russo M, Dono F, et al. Agitation and Dementia: Prevention and Treatment Strategies in Acute and Chronic Conditions. *Frontiers in Neurology*. 2021;12. doi:https://doi.org/10.3389/fneur.2021.644317

2. *Oxford Textbook of Palliative Medicine*. Oxford Univ Press; 2021

3. Tieges Z, Maclullich AMJ, Anand A, et al. Diagnostic accuracy of the 4AT for delirium detection in older adults: systematic review and meta-analysis. *Age Ageing*. 2021;50(3):733-743. doi:10.1093/ageing/afaa224

4. Rosen J, Burgio L, Kollar M, et al. The Pittsburgh Agitation Scale: A User-Friendly Instrument for Rating Agitation in Dementia Patients. *Am J Geriatr Psychiatry*. 1994;2(1):52-59. doi:10.1097/00019442-199400210-00008

5. Code of Federal Regulations Title 42 Chapter IV Subchapter B Part 418 Hospice Care. National Archives and Records Administration.https://www.ecfr.gov/current/title-42/chapter-IV/subchapter-B/part-418 Accessed June 5, 2023

Further Reading:

Heldt JP. *Memorable Psychopharmacology*. Createspace Independent Publishing Platform; 2021.

24.
Hospice Program Quality Measures

> *An idea, like a ghost, must be spoken to a little before it will explain itself.*
>
> Charles Dickens

As a federal entitlement program, there are metrics that CMS uses to measure the quality of the hospice care provided. As part of an interdisciplinary team, you should realize that your care and that of your team will impact the quality of care provided, as well as the perception by patients and their families. Ultimately your care will be scored.

The Hospice Quality Reporting Program (HQRP) uses data to calculate the quality of the performance on quality measures provided by your hospice program.

Table 9 summarizes four of the measures CMS is looking at to judge the quality of care your hospice program is delivering. Your entire team should be aware that care is being measured. I recommend working with your Quality Improvement director and being aware of the gaps your program faces and potential areas of improvement that can be worked on as quality improvement projects.

Table 9. Hospice Quality Reporting Program Measures Summary [1].

HIS Comprehensive Assessment Measure at Admission	It will measure the proportion of patients where the hospice performed all seven of the care process measured.
HVLDL	Measures the proportion of patients that received in-person visits from a registered nurse or a medical social worker in the last 3 days of life.
Hospice Care Index	It is a single measure calculated from ten indicators
CAHPS Hospice Survey	Measures caregiver perception of the care provided to the patient after they have expired.

I will add a little snippet from each one of the above measures and give you my take. I am including the link to the page that provides more details on the hospice quality measures CMS reviews in the references [1]. On the left-hand side of the reference page, you will find the column with all the specific links to each one of these quality measures [1].

The HIS measures are important quality indicators of clinical hospice care. Five of these measures deal with symptoms. Two address pain, and two address dyspnea. One addresses opioid-induced constipation.

Measure Description:	The HIS Comprehensive Assessment at Admission (NQF #3235) captures, in a single measure, the proportion of patients for whom the hospice performed all seven care processes, as applicable. The care processes include: 1. Beliefs/Values Addressed (if desired by the patient) 2. Treatment Preferences 3. Pain Screening 4. Pain Assessment 5. Dyspnea Treatment 6. Dyspnea Screening 7. Patients Treated with an Opioid who are Given a Bowel Regimen

Figure 9. Hospice and Palliative Care Composite Process Measure- HIS Comprehensive Assessment at Admission[2].

Let's look at an example.

Mr. Lee is a 75-year-old patient admitted to hospice 7 days ago with metastatic prostate cancer. He had uncontrolled pain. He was determined to be opioid naïve and was placed on Methadone 2.5 mg p.o. q 12 hours with immediate-release morphine release 5 mg q 4 hours prn for breakthrough pain. You call to follow up, and his daughter informs you her Dad appears much more comfortable and can tolerate the pain. She is though concerned because he has not had a bowel movement.

Did you forget something? Look at the HIS measures above in Figure 9. These are all important, but I want to call your attention to #7. Any patient who is started on an opioid needs a bowel regimen (laxative). This is an essential primary palliative intervention! You would be surprised at how this can be missed. Make sure you provide laxities to any hospice patient on opioids.

The link in the references will take you to the HIS measure page. There are several manuals in pdf that you can access and print out if you want more details about these specific measures [2].

Another metric you and the hospice team must pay attention to is the Hospice Visits in the Last Days of Life. I will stress again the importance of recognizing when a patient may be imminent. Recall we reviewed how this is important for families. Guess what? It is a CMS quality measure. Your prognostication skills are being measured.

Measure Description:	The HVLDL measure assesses hospice staff visits to patients at the end of life. This measure is constructed from Medicare hospice claims records. It indicates the hospice provider's proportion of patients who have received in-person visits from a registered nurse or medical social worker on at least two out of the final three days of the patient's life. Note: The last three days are defined as: (Day 1) the day of death, (Day 2) the day prior to death, and (Day 3) the day two days prior to death.

Figure 10. Hospice Visits in Last Days of Life (HVLDL) [1].

Caregivers of hospice patients most appreciate a visit from their RN and the social worker when the patient is imminent. The visit by all the members of the interdisciplinary team is important; it is, however, the RN and social worker's visits which are reported as a quality measure to CMS (Fig.10). Your team should take the opportunity at the IDG meeting to discuss patients who may be imminent. You should review with your team continuously how to identify an imminent patient. It can improve your quality scores, but most importantly, provide the proper support for patients and families during a critical end-of-life period.

The Hospice Care Index looks at different events that occur to patients throughout their hospice stay (Fig 11).

Measure Description:	The Hospice Care Index (HCI) captures care processes occurring throughout the hospice stay, between admission and discharge. The HCI is a single measure comprising ten indicators calculated from Medicare claims data. The indicators included in the HCI are listed below this table. The index design of the HCI simultaneously monitors all ten indicators. Collectively these indicators represent different aspects of hospice service and thereby characterize hospices comprehensively, rather than on just a single care dimension. Each indicator equally affects the single HCI score, reflecting the equal importance of each aspect of care delivered from admission to discharge.

Figure 11. Hospice Care Index (HCI) [1].

- What are these measures?

1. Continuous Home Care (CHC) or General Inpatient (GIP) Provided
2. Gaps in Skilled Nursing Visits
3. Early Live Discharges
4. Late Live Discharges
5. Burdensome Transitions (Type 1) – Live Discharges from Hospice Followed by Hospitalization and Subsequent Hospice Readmission
6. Burdensome Transitions (Type 2) – Live Discharges from Hospice Followed by Hospitalization with the Patient Dying in the Hospital
7. Per-beneficiary Medicare Spending
8. Skilled Nursing Care Minutes per Routine Home Care (RHC) Day
9. Skilled Nursing Minutes on Weekends
10. Visits Near Death

As you can see, there are several things that you, as a physician, play a key role in. Are you able to justify why you are ordering continuous care? Are you providing a clear rationale for what is being addressed and how the patient responds to the intervention? What about the GIP level of care? Is it being used appropriately? Are patients revoking hospice and being readmitted to the hospital? Did they understand where they were in their disease trajectory? Do you understand why I keep stating to use the disease trajectory graphs (Fig.2) to emphasize end-of-life to your patients and families? Notice that # 10 takes into account the visits near death. Are you and your team assessing your patients to identify imminent patients? Are the RN and social worker visiting imminent patients?

References

1. Current Measures. Centers for Medicare & Medicaid Services CMS.gov https://www.cms.gov/Medicare/Quality-Initiatives-Patient-Assessment-Instruments/Hospice-Quality-Reporting/Current-Measures Accessed June 25, 2023.

2. Hospice Item Set (HIS) Centers for Medicare & Medicaid Services. CMS.gov https://www.cms.gov/Medicare/Quality-Initiatives-Patient-Assessment-Instruments/Hospice-Quality-Reporting/Hospice-Item-Set-HIS Accessed June 25, 2023

25.
Consumer Assessment of Healthcare Providers and Systems (CAHPS®) Hospice Survey

> *True independence and freedom can only exist in doing what's right.*
> Brigham Young

Yes, just like hospitals and outpatient clinic practices, we also have a patient experience score for hospice! CMS started work on this survey tool in 2012. Before the CAHPS hospice survey, there was no way to measure a patient and/or family's experience with hospice care. The first public reporting of this survey occurred in 2018. Unlike the other patient experience surveys, the CAHPS is sent to the patient's officially documented primary care provider two months after the patient has expired. The primary care provider has 42 days to complete and return the survey. The purpose of the survey is to allow to obtain objective and meaningful comparisons of hospice providers. It serves as an incentive for hospices to improve their quality of care [1].

CMS is looking at [2]:

1. Communication with family
2. Access to timely help
3. Treating patients with respect (Just like the other surveys)
4. Emotional and spiritual support
5. Help for pain and symptom management Training Family to Care for Patients
6. Rating of the Hospice program
7. Willing to Recommend Hospice program

All of these are essential and are a way for caregivers to provide feedback on the perceived quality of care your hospice team provides to their loved ones. I want you to look at number #5. This helps to cement the importance of the expertise you bring to your hospice team as a physician. You need to bring your A-game when it comes to pain and symptom management.

You will not likely remember all of the details of these measures, but you need to be aware that they exist. They are measures used by CMS, and as a hospice physician, you will impact some of them. As part of a hospice interdisciplinary team, you will impact all of them.

You do share responsibility on your hospice programs well-being and ability to continue to operate. If for no other reason to ensure that high quality care can continue to be provided to patients and families in your community. Recall that CMS is still working on tying quality measures to hospice care provisions. There quality reporting measures will impact the Hospice Wage Index.

It takes a team of dedicated individuals to deliver a holistic, interdisciplinary team-based approach. Hospice care is complex, but it does not have to be complicated as long as you work as part of an interdisciplinary team.

References

1. CAHPS Hospice Survey. Quality Assurance Guidelines. Version 7.0 September 2020.

2. CAHPS Hospice Survey. CMS.gov. https://www.cms.gov/Medicare/Quality-Initiatives-Patient-Assessment-Instruments/Hospice-Quality-Reporting/CAHPS%C2%AE-Hospice-Survey Accessed June 25, 2023

26.

The Elephant in the Room: Medical Assistance in Dying (MAiD)

> *If a man could have half of his wishes, he would double his troubles.*
> Benjamin Franklin

Mrs. Doe is a 77-year-old female patient with end-stage heart failure. She is noticeably cachectic and is not able to speak in full sentences. She is using accessory muscles and her speech is garbled. You are assessing her and determining that morphine should be provided to help manage her evident dyspnea and discomfort. You discuss your plan with her daughter who is her proxy. She asks if you could provide more morphine to help her mother pass away and not have to suffer anymore.

How would you respond?

Irrespective of your personal belief and views on Medical Aid in Dying (MAiD), we do not endorse euthanasia in hospice! Read again. As a federal entitlement program, we abide by the Assisted Suicide Funding Restriction Act (ASFRA) passed in 1997 which essentially states that federal funding MAY NOT BE USED to cause, or assist in causing the death of an individual by suicide ASFRA, 1997 14404(a)(1). A hospice provider would lose their funding if they were determined to willfully participated in MAiD [1].

As a hospice physician, it is therefore of the utmost importance to be explicit and deliberate to explain and document your intent. It should be clear that prescribing any of the medications we commonly use with a narrow therapeutic index is for symptom management. Any intervention provided should be with the sole purpose of addressing and alleviating distressing symptoms at end-of-life.

What if you practice in a State where MAiD is permitted and legal? Again we do not provide MAiD in Medicare-certified hospices! Why? FEDERAL LAW would supersede any State law based on the concept of supremacy where the more stringent form of the law prevails!

MAiD would not be necessary for a patient to contemplate if we can ensure that we can provide equitable, timely, high-quality end-of-life palliative care through hospice. I am painfully aware that we are far from ideal access to hospice care. MAiD should not be the only choice a patient perceives to have due to lack of access to hospice. If we want patients to have a choice and voice in their end-of-life care, we need to continue to work to ensure equitable access to hospice. Hospice care needs to be inclusive and respect and celebrate diversity. When we advocate and work towards these ideals, we are inherently working towards promoting social justice.

When addressing hospice interventions, especially medications, remember to educate patients and families on intent and proportionality. Document your conversations.

I will leave an excellent resource for you to expand on ethics at end-of-life under further reading.

Reference

1. H.R 1003 Assisted Suicide Funding Restriction Act of 1997. Congress.Gov. https://www.congress.gov/bill/105th-congress/house-bill/1003 Accessed July 12, 2023

Further Reading:

Macauley RC. *Ethics in Palliative Care : A Complete guide*. Oxford University Press; 2018.

27.
Death Certificates

The wise does at once what the fool does at last.

Baltasar Gracian

You will be asked to sign death certificates as a hospice physician. Is it the responsibility of a hospice physician to sign them? Allow me to share some insights on this topic. A death certificate is the final page in a human being's journey. A birth certificate is one bookend; the death certificate is the other. Death certificates allow us to contribute to studying disease prevalence in the U.S. when you accurately complete them. We can better understand morbidity and mortality trends. Most importantly, bereaved family members are dealing with grief at the passing of their loved one and need the death certificate to be completed promptly. Burial or cremation cannot move forward until the death certificate is completed. Family members require a completed death certificate to access accounts, pay bills, transfer funds, and legally close accounts. Providing a timely complete death certificate allows the family to progress in their grieving process [1].

What if the patient was on hospice for a short stay and cannot access their detailed records? You should try your best to obtain or review any available records in a reasonable time to complete the death certificate. There should be a space on the certificate to list other significant conditions. This is where I add the following: HOSPICE PATIENT, TERMINALLY ILL. If there are no records or they are limited and do not allow me to be specific, I will also add on the same line: LIMITED MEDICAL RECORDS.

Here is an example of a patient who was admitted to hospice with a primary diagnosis of cerebral atherosclerosis. Here is how I would complete the death certificate. Note that cerebral atherosclerosis is not listed as the immediate cause. Long-standing essential hypertension causes shearing to the endothelium. The body repairs these shears by depositing cholesterol which in turn causes irregularities in the arterial vasculature, impairing the flow of blood and increasing propensity to clot formations. In essence, this is what leads to cerebral atherosclerosis (Atherosclerosis affects all the arteries not just the ones in the brain). As a consequence, the patient develops vascular dementia, and as time goes by due to a lack of normal blood supply the brain shrinks and we arrive at cerebral atrophy.

Image 2. Death Certificate Example.

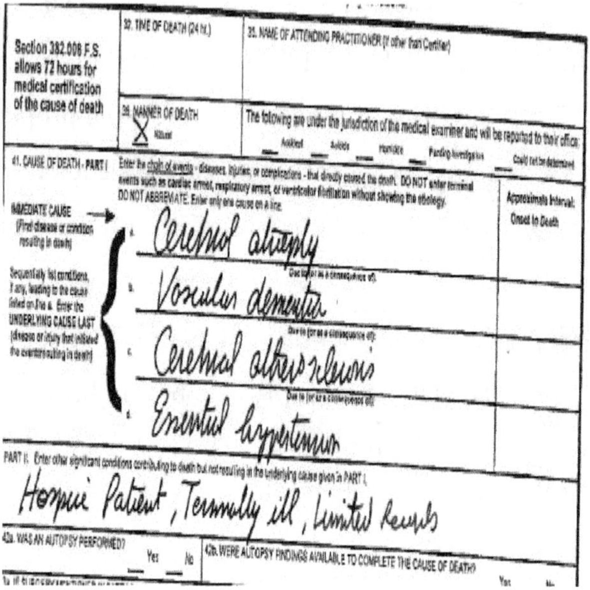
Section 382.008 F.S. allows 72 hours for medical certification of the cause of death

32. TIME OF DEATH (24 hr.)

35. NAME OF ATTENDING PRACTITIONER (If other than Certifier)

38. MANNER OF DEATH

X Natural

The following are under the jurisdiction of the medical examiner and will be reported to their office:

_ Accident _ Suicide _ Homicide _ Pending Investigation _ Could not be determined

41. CAUSE OF DEATH - PART I

Enter the chain of events - diseases, injuries, or complications - that directly caused the death. DO NOT enter terminal events such as cardiac arrest, respiratory arrest, or ventricular fibrillation without showing the etiology. DO NOT ABBREVIATE. Enter only one cause on a line.

Approximate Interval: Onset to Death

IMMEDIATE CAUSE (Final disease or condition resulting in death)

Sequentially list conditions, if any, leading to the cause listed on line a. Enter the UNDERLYING CAUSE LAST (disease or injury that initiated the events resulting in death)

a. Cerebral atrophy

Due to (or as a consequence of):

b. Vascular dementia

Due to (or as a consequence of):

c. Cerebral atherosclerosis

Due to (or as a consequence of):

d. Essential hypertension

PART II. Enter other significant conditions contributing to death but not resulting in the underlying cause given in PART I.

Hospice Patient, Terminally ill, Limited Results

42a. WAS AN AUTOPSY PERFORMED? _ Yes _ No

42b. WERE AUTOPSY FINDINGS AVAILABLE TO COMPLETE THE CAUSE OF DEATH? Yes No

Let's look at another example where the patient was admitted to hospice while in the hospital and expired in the hospital under GIP 24 hours later.

Image 3. Death Certificate Example.

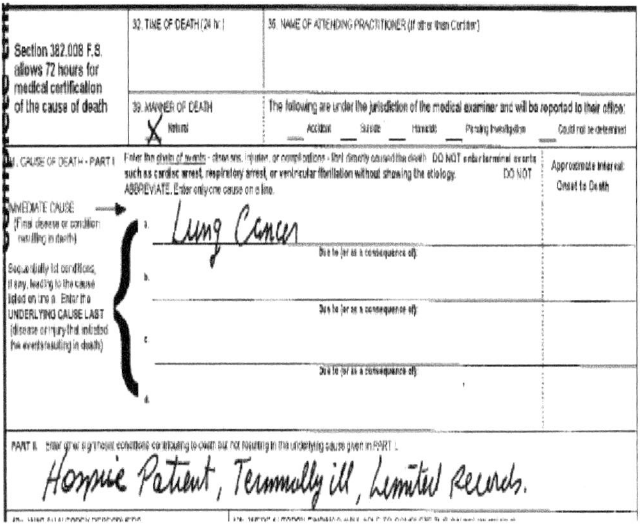
Section 382.008 F.S. allows 72 hours for medical certification of the cause of death

32. TIME OF DEATH (24 hr.)

36. NAME OF ATTENDING PRACTITIONER (If other than Certifier)

39. MANNER OF DEATH

X Natural

The following are under the jurisdiction of the medical examiner and will be reported to their office:

__ Accident __ Suicide __ Homicide __ Pending Investigation __ Could not be determined

41. CAUSE OF DEATH - PART I Enter the chain of events - diseases, injuries, or complications - that directly caused the death. DO NOT enter terminal events such as cardiac arrest, respiratory arrest, or ventricular fibrillation without showing the etiology. DO NOT ABBREVIATE. Enter only one cause on a line.

Approximate Interval: Onset to Death

IMMEDIATE CAUSE (Final disease or condition resulting in death) → a. Lung Cancer

Due to (or as a consequence of):

Sequentially list conditions, if any, leading to the cause listed on line a. Enter the UNDERLYING CAUSE LAST (disease or injury that initiated the events resulting in death)

b.

Due to (or as a consequence of):

c.

Due to (or as a consequence of):

d.

PART II. Enter other significant conditions contributing to death but not resulting in the underlying cause given in PART I.

Hospice Patient, Terminally ill, Limited Records.

I was sent the above death certificate to sign however the primary diagnosis listed in our hospice case sheet was “Malignancy unspecified, other”. You cannot use malignancy unspecified and if you do expect the Medical Examiner to reject the certificate. I had to spend a bit of time going through the scant records that were available, and I was able to find that the patient had lung cancer. I would have preferred to document the type of lung cancer, laterality, or if it was metastatic. Unfortunately, these details were not available. Adding "limited records" was a recommendation provided to me by my Medical Examiner's office. This allows the Medical Examiner to know that I did the best I could with the limited information made available when the death certificate was completed. I recommend you contact your local Medical Examiner's office and introduce yourself. Keep their contact handy, as there will be cases requiring further review with them.

I have found the book by Dr. Erica Armstrong to be an excellent guide and reference. Reading the book will clarify how pathologists think and why death certificates need to be completed a certain way, such as in the examples I provided. I highly recommend having a copy and referencing it for completing death certificates [1].

Reference

1. Armstrong EJ. *Essentials of Death Reporting and Death Certification*. Erica Armstrong; 2017.

28.

Bereavement and Condolences

> *The whole is more than the sum of its parts.*
>
> Aristotle

42 CFR 418.54(c)(7)[1] speaks about the initial bereavement assessment that must be completed at admission. This assessment focuses on the needs of the patient's family and other individuals close to the patient, with attention to the social, spiritual, and cultural factors that may impact their ability to cope with the patient's death. 42 CFR 418.204(c)[1] states that bereavement counseling is a required hospice service but is not reimbursable. As per 42 CFR 418.64(d)(1)(ii)[1], bereavement is to be provided for 12 months after a patient has died. By convention, all hospice providers

provide bereavement for 13 months so as to not end the support to the family and those close to the patient on the anniversary of their passing. This important service is not reimbursed. It is factored into the total Medicare spending for the time hospice provided care to the patient. Once again when you read those amazing sensational headlines about the multibillion-dollar hospice industry, you will likely never read about how care, yes care is still being provided by the hospice team after the patient has passed away.

Writing a condolence note to a family member who has just lost a loved one is difficult, but it serves as a heartfelt gesture of sympathy and support during a difficult time of loss. Expressing condolences through a written note allows you to reach out to the grieving family and provide comfort and solace. Your chaplain will likely initiate a condolence card for the team to sign. Signing the condolence cards is good practice and part of being an excellent interdisciplinary team member. Families do notice and do appreciate the gesture. I am very fortunate to work with an amazing hospice team, and among my teammates, the team chaplain initiates bereavement services for the family and calls the primary caregiver on behalf of the team to express condolences. If you as the physician know the primary caregiver and family, it is always good practice to call yourself and give your condolences.

Reference

1. Code of Federal Regulations Title 42 Chapter IV Subchapter B Part 418 Hospice Care. National Archives and Records Administration.https://www.ecfr.gov/current/title-42/chapter-IV/subchapter-B/part-418 Accessed June 5, 2023

Further Reading:

Isaacs F. *My Deepest Sympathies...* Potter Style; 2010.

29.
Hospice Advocacy in the Community

> *Remember upon the conduct of each depends the fate of all.*
> Alexander The Great

Hospice advocacy is vital in ensuring compassionate and quality end-of-life care for patients and families. Being an engaged advocate allows for the removal of barriers to equitable hospice access.

Here are some talking points you may want to consider as you go into the community and advocate for hospice. These will likely be the questions fellow healthcare clinicians not aware of hospice may ask as well as questions that patients and their families will have for you as a hospice physician.

1. **Hospice means giving up.**

   We can explain the care that an eligible patient and their family are expected to receive. The key point here is to share that we do not stop caring, we just change gears on how we care. Patients and families are usually amazed at the number of resources they are provided once they enroll in hospice.

2. **You need a clinician to refer you to hospice.**

   As an entitlement program, anyone can elect to be evaluated. The point we want to make here is that clinicians do not determine that a patient must transition to hospice because there is nothing left to do. The physician's role is simply to determine if a patient is at the point in their disease trajectory that they are now eligible to receive their hospice benefit.

3. **Hospice enrollment means a patient no longer has a say in their care.**

Patient and their families are considered integral parts of the care team and their input is necessary to create an individualized plan of care unique to the patient and their specific needs at end-of-life.

4. Once signed on to hospice you must remain in hospice.

As an entitlement program, patients have the right to revoke their Medicare hospice benefit at any time. Often, we have patients revoking hospice to return to the hospital only to find that the interventions offered can also be comfortably provided by hospice. This is a crucial point to educate patients and families on. The disease trajectory does not reverse itself and the interventions offered outside of hospice do not decrease mortality or improve prognosis.

5. Hospice is expensive

Hospice is 100% covered. Medicare Part A becomes hospice and there are no copays or deductibles.

Interdisciplinary care team services, equipment such as hospital beds, and medications in use for terminal conditions symptom management are completely covered with no out-of-pocket cost for patients and families.

6. Hospice is only for the patient.

Hospice is holistic care for patients and their immediate families. As an example of a benefit for families, bereavement services are provided for 13 months after their loved one passes away.

7. Hospice and palliative care are the same things.

There is a lot of confusion about hospice and palliative care. All hospice care is palliative care yet not all palliative care is hospice. The philosophical underpinnings are the same, however, hospice is covered as a federal program. Palliative care is funded as a Fee for Service (FFE) specialty and is not present in all U.S. hospitals. Most palliative care services lack the necessary support structure for patients to receive home-based care. Patients and families are not likely to know the differences, especially as far as the support provided. As we continue to evolve in our healthcare delivery we need to expand palliative care services to the community outside of acute care settings as well as look into ways to incorporate palliative care into the hospice benefit and provide services much sooner in a patient's disease process.

8. You must have a DNR to elect hospice.

DNR is never required. A federal entitlement program cannot be based on code status. The interdisciplinary hospice team will explore the rationale for code status and clarify any misunderstandings with patients and families.

9. Hospice is only for six months.

The initial certification is for the provision of service for six months. If a beneficiary reaches the six-month threshold they can be recertified for another two months as long as we can show a progressive decline in either functionality, nutrition, or cognition. We can continue to recertify indefinitely every two months as long as there is continued decline.

10. Hospice is a physical place.

Hospice is provided wherever the patient calls home while in other countries patients go to hospice. We should highlight this unique difference.

11. Hospice is only for cancer.

Hospice is for any patient that has a chronic progressive terminal disease and they have reached the end-stage of the disease process.

12. If I choose hospice, I will lose my primary care physician.

PCPs are considered to be integral members of the hospice team. They can remain as active in the care plan as they choose to be and can participate in the hospice plan of care.

13. If I elect hospice, they will stop all medications.

Medications will be reviewed with patients and families and they will be educated on the lack of benefits at this stage of their life. A clear rationale will be provided as to why any particular medication should be stopped and it will be a shared decision. Medications are never automatically stopped at the time of hospice enrollment.

14. If I am in hospice, I cannot go to the hospital.

Should a beneficiary require care above what can be provided in the comfort of their home to stabilize symptoms, hospice will transfer them for a short period to one of their inpatient units if doing so aligns with patients' preferences.

15. Morphine will be given to expedite a patient's demise.

No intervention will ever be provided by the hospice to expedite a patient's demise! Hospice will support the natural dying process and focus on providing the optimal quality of life for whatever time is remaining. Opioids such as morphine are only used to alleviate pain and the doses used are proportional to the patient's needs.

It will take all of us to raise awareness about hospice care. The more we educate, the sooner we allow patients and their families to access their hospice benefit and allow them to complete their life journey with grace, respect, and dignity while receiving holistic interdisciplinary care and support at end-of-life.

30.
Final Thoughts

My intent here was to give you an overall picture of practicing as a non- Hospice and Palliative Medicine trained hospice physician and share some of the complexities you will need to navigate. Hopefully, this will stimulate your curiosity and you will keep learning more about hospice care, and advocate for its quality. Providing the financial facts was to show you that your clinical decisions may impact the well-being of your hospice program and the care your patients and families receive.

I leave you with these final thoughts:

1. Human beings are mortal

2. Technology cannot correct biology. We have not found a way to cure the progression of biological decline. We discover new ways to support the aging body but these interventions will not restore youth. Remember the disease trajectory graphs at the beginning of this guide.

3. Hospice is a part of Medicare and is intended for patients who have reached the terminal phase of their disease. It can also be provided to end-of-life patients outside of Medicare through Medicaid, private insurance, and charity care.

4. Present hospice as the benefit as it is, emphasizing it is the patient's choice.

5. Familiarize yourself with the Code of Federal Regulations Title 42 Part 418. It spells out the hospice regulations or conditions of participation.

6. Continue to learn and grow. Read, read, read. Seek out opportunities to learn about hospice and palliative care.

7. Consider becoming board certified in hospice. If you want to provide quality end-of-life care to patients and families, you will also want to be recognized for your expertise and commitment to end-of-life care. Take the Hospice Medical Director Certification (HMDC) exam. It is for all physicians practicing hospice and not just for physicians serving in hospice administrator roles. https://hmdcb.org/

8. Not everyone can provide end-of-life care. Be proud to make a difference.

9. You are not alone! You are part of an interdisciplinary care team. Respect your team members and rely on their skills. They will complement yours and make it possible to provide the best possible care to patients and families at end-of-life.

10. Hospice is about quality of life at end-of-life. That is our ethos!

Index

acute-short-term hospitals, 15
admission, 90
Advance Care Directives, 36
advance care planning, 33
Advance Care Planning, 36
advance directive, 33
Advanced Practice Registered Nurse, 93
Affordable Care Act, 22
Agitation, 177
amyotrophic lateral disease, 21
anticoagulation, 155
Anxiety, 128
arterial blood gas, 102
Artificial Nutrition and Hydration, 39
Assisted Suicide Funding Restriction Act, 196
benzodiazepines, 180
bereavement assessment, 205
billing modifiers, 161
CAHPS, 191
Cancer, 85
care flow chart, 155
Caregiver breakdown, 132
Centers for Medicare and Medicaid, 74
cerebral atherosclerosis, 92
certification narrative, 92
certification period, 92
certified, 80
chronic progressive terminal disease, 26, 47
Cicely Saunders, 10
Clinical Judgement, 99
clinical judgment, 84
CMS, 81
Code of Federal Regulations, 79, 98
codified, 79
cognition, 65
comprehensive assessment, 90, 91
Conditions of Participation, 80
condolence note, 206
Congestive Heart Failure, 85
Constipation, 128
Continuous home care, 131
Conversation Guide, 40

COPD, 85
Cor Pulmonale, 102
crucial conversation, 51
death certificate, 198
death-denying culture, 26
Dementia, 85
dialysis, 21, 23, 24
Disabling dyspnea at rest, 100
discharge for cause, 116
Discharge from Hospice, 109
disease trajectory, 27, 44
disease-directed care, 48
Disease-directed treatment, 108
DNR, 25
Do not hospitalize, 38
Do not resuscitate order (DNR), 37
doctor of medicine, 120
Durable power of attorney for health care, 37
Eastern Cooperative Oncology Group, 61
ECHO, 102
ECOG, 76
eligible, 80
Elizabeth Kübler Ross, 11
Emergency Department, 17
emotional, 91
entitlement program, 49

face-to-face, 89, 93
Fast Facts Palliative Care Network of Wisconsin, 173
federal entitlement program, 104
fentanyl patch, 169
Fiscal Year, 143
Florance Wald, 11
functionality, 65
General inpatient care, 134
General Inpatient level, 84
HIS measures, 185
Hospice Care Index, 188
hospice eligible, 46
Hospice Medical Director Certification (HMDC) exam, 217
hospice physician, 40
Hospice Quality Reporting Program, 183
hospice survey, 191
Hospice Visits in the Last Days of Life, 187
Hospice Wage Index, 142
Hospices, 10
Hospital Survey and Construction Act of 1946, 14
hospital-centric healthcare, 14
Hypoxia, 101
ICU, 33
IDG, 53

224

imminence, 71
imminent, 70
initial 90 days, 81
interdisciplinary group, 121
Interdisciplinary Group, 71
Intervention, 172
Karnofsky Performance Scale, 55
laboratory monitoring, 125
Living Will, 37
local coverage determinations, 97
Local Coverage Determinations, *86*
median survival, 66, 73
Medicaid, 82
Medical Aid in Dying (MAiD), 196
Medical orders for life-sustaining treatment, 39
Medicare Administrative Contractor, 96
Medicare Administrative Contractors, 85
Medicare Advantage, 19
Medicare deductibles, 160
Medicare Hospice Benefit, 82
Medicare Modernization Act, 19
Medicare Part A, 20, 139
Medicare Part D, 127

medication-relatedness, 126
medications, 31, 124
National Institute of Aging, 39
Nausea, 128
network, 96
NHPCO, 127
notice of election, 82
notice of termination, 118
nutrition, 65
opioid-naïve, 166
opioid-tolerant, 166
osteopathy, 120
Outcome, 173
Pain, 128
Palliative Care service, 52
Palliative Performance Score, 55
Patient Self-Determination Act, 34
peripheral cyanosis, 71
physical, 91
physician, 120
Physician orders for life-sustaining treatment, 39
physician workforce, 16
pill burden, 124
plateau, 77
PPS, 76
preferences, 32
preventive measure, 126

225

primary care physicians, 17
Primary care physicians, 159
prognosis, 87
Prognostication funnel, 77
prognostication., 75
proxy, 33
psychosocial, 91
pulmonary embolism, 154
Quality Improvement, 184
Quick Flip, 105
rehabilitation, 20
RELATED, 153
Respite care, 133
revoke, 106
Right heart failure, 101
Routine home care, 129
side effects, 124
Skilled Nursing Facilities, 20
specialists, 16

SPIKES protocol, 47
spiritual, 91
subsequent 90 days, 81
systemic review, 164
tachycardia, 101
Tax Equity and Fiscal Responsibility Act of 1982, 12
technology-driven care, 16
terminal prognosis, 125
tools, 67
uncontrolled symptoms, 151
Unintentional progressive weight loss, 101
UNRELATED, 153
Utilization Medical Director, 83
Volunteer services, 122
wishes and values, 32
written certification, 81

I hope you found this short guide helpful.

Questions or comments can be directed to:

andy.arwari@gmail.com